WB 4

D0551396

PHYSIOTHERAPY AND THE ELDERLY PATIENT

THERAPY IN PRACTICE
Series Editor: Jo Campling

This series of books is aimed at 'therapists' concerned with rehabilitation in a very broad sense. The intended audience particularly includes occupational therapists, physiotherapists and speech therapists, but many titles will also be of interest to nurses, psychologists, medical staff, social workers, teachers or volunteer workers. Some volumes will be interdisciplinary, others aimed at one particular profession. All titles will be comprehensive but concise, and practical but with due reference to relevant theory and evidence. They are not research monographs but focus on professional practice, and will be of value to both students and qualified personnel.

Physiotherapy and the Elderly Patient

PAUL WAGSTAFF
M.A. M.Sc. M.C.S.P. Grad. Dip. Phys. Dip.T.P.
Director and Senior Lecturer
School of Physiotherapy
Trinity College, Dublin

and

DAVIS COAKLEY
M.D. F.R.C.P.I.
Professor of Geriatric Medicine and
Director of Postgraduate Medical Education
Trinity College, Dublin
and
Consultant Physician
St. James's Hospital, Dublin

CROOM HELM
London & Sydney

© 1988 Paul Wagstaff and Davis Coakley
Croom Helm Ltd, Provident House,
Burrell Row, Beckenham, Kent BR3 1AT

Croom Helm Australia, 44–50 Waterloo Road,
North Ryde, 2113, New South Wales

British Library Cataloguing in Publication Data

Wagstaff, Paul
  Physiotherapy and the elderly patient.
  — (Therapy in practice).
  1. Geriatrics 2. Physical therapy
  I. Title   II. Coakley, Davis   III. Series
  618.97   RC953.5

  ISBN 0-7099-3696-6

Filmset by Mayhew Typesetting, Bristol, England
Printed and bound in Great Britain by
Biddles Ltd, Guildford and King's Lynn

Contents

Preface

There is a growing awareness of the importance of the specialty of the care of elderly people and the need for physiotherapists to be familiar with its precepts, since almost all of them will spend a good deal of their time treating older patients. The aim of this book is to introduce the physiotherapy student and the clinical physiotherapist to the multifaceted components involved in the care of elderly patients and to present a problem-oriented approach to assessment and management.

Recent years have seen the gradual emergence of a more positive approach to the problems of the elderly. The introduction of the specialty to the undergraduate course at the School of Physiotherapy, Trinity College, Dublin, where both the authors teach, has provided an impetus for research and investigation into physiotherapy of the elderly patient. The series of lectures, seminars, tutorials and clinical experience, which students receive, extends from the second to the fourth year. In the final year, a specialist option in the area can be undertaken. The purpose of this option is to enable the student to develop a more comprehensive knowledge of the subject. As a result of these developments, several research projects have been undertaken at both student and staff levels. The specialty has received far greater emphasis than was the case in former years and the course bears a closer relationship to the realities of current practice and the needs of the community.

It is hoped that this book, as well as acting as a practical manual, will stimulate both students and clinicians to question current rehabilitation and physiotherapy practices. In this way, therapy skills and attitudes will continue to improve. Care of elderly people will demand the dynamic and responsible approach so necessary for achievement in this area. The frustrations and disillusionments of the past will be overcome and the patient, who is after all the ultimate aim of the endeavour, will receive better treatment and care.

Acknowledgements

We wish to thank Professor Eamon Sweeney for the illustrations in Figure 4.2, 5.1–4, 6.1, 8.1–2 and 15.1; Mrs G. McGowan for Figures 7.1 and 7.2; Mr David Smith for the photographs in Figures 6.2 and 6.3 and Mr Michael Cummins for the photograph in Figure 11.1. Figure 3.1 was designed by Ms Ann Finn of the School of Physiotherapy, University of Dublin. We would also like to thank her for her enthusiastic development of the course on the elderly in the School of Physiotherapy.

We would also like to thank Joan Kealy, Senior Physiotherapist at St James's Hospital, for reading and commenting on sections of the book during its presentation. Our wives Sandy Wagstaff and Mary Coakley gave us considerable practical help with the work at various stages and we are also very grateful to them for their encouragement throughout. We would also like to acknowledge the help of our secretaries Lilian Stanbridge and Mary Clarke.

Finally we would like to thank Tim Hardwick of Croom Helm for his interest and support.

1

Growing Old

The absolute number of elderly people in western society has increased dramatically during this century. At present, the average proportion of elderly people i.e. throughout the world is around 4 per cent, whereas in Europe, the average is about 14 per cent. This phenomenon has been described as 'the greying of nations'. In the 40-year span between 1931 and 1971, the number of people aged 65 and over in England and Wales doubled in number from about 3 million to over 6 million. Even more significantly, the number of people who are very old, i.e. aged 75 and over, trebled from 800,000 to 2,400,000. This increase in the proportion of elderly people in the population, including the number of very frail elderly, is predicted to continue in England and Wales for the next 20 years.

Another important feature in the ageing of the population is the differential between males and females. For instance, the females born this year in France are expected to outlive their male companions by 8 years (Paillat 1981). Physiotherapists working in a department of geriatric medicine will quickly realise that the majority of their patients are female. It is a common error to assume that the increased proportion of elderly people in our population is due to advances in medical care since World War II. In fact, it is due to the fall in childhood mortality that was the result of better social conditions towards the end of the last century and the beginning of this century. More children survived to grow into young adults and now these young adults are growing old.

Morbidity (the rate of illness) rises steeply with age. It is extremely high in patients over the age of 75 and these patients are also referred to as the 'old old'. Although they account for only 14 per cent of the population in the UK, elderly patients occupy over 50 per cent of hospital beds. If the demand for institutional care is to be controlled in the future, there must be some radical rethinking in society's approach to old age. The physiotherapist has a key role in planning such new approaches. A more determined effort must be made to keep elderly people independent and healthy in old age. Only in this way will the demand for institutional care diminish. Physiotherapists can assist not only by treating individual patients and enabling them to become more mobile and independent, but also by becoming involved in educating groups on how to remain healthy and active in old age. This educational process must begin before retirement. They can also help in fostering a more positive attitude to older people, both in hospital and in the community.

ATTITUDES TOWARDS ELDERLY PEOPLE

If any programme for the elderly is going to succeed, the attitudes of the professional people involved must be right. In general, attitudes towards the elderly in society tend to be negative. In an era where technological skills are priced above all else, knowledge of traditional skills handed down from generation to generation has lost its value. Respect for age has changed in many places to frank prejudice against age. The stereotype of ageing is one of illness, fatigue, disinterest in sexual affairs and intellectual dullness (McTavish 1971). However, these stereotyped attitudes are often linked to socio-economic factors, as attitudes towards old people who are educated, healthy and affluent can be quite different.

An American survey found that the interest of medical students in the problems of the elderly diminished as their undergraduate course progressed. Part of the decline in interest was thought to be due to the negative attitude of educators and more positive attitudes were found in students exposed to a high standard of teaching in the medicine of old age (National Academy of Sciences 1978). Rowlings (1981) acknowledged that social workers may have deep-seated prejudices about old age. Similarly, Mills (1972) found that American occupational therapy students were deficient in their knowledge of the ageing process and in general were not interested in working with geriatric patients. Peach (1978) found similar negative attitudes in a study involving the final-year students in eight schools of physiotherapy in Britain.

Finn (1986) studied the attitudes of practising physiotherapists towards geriatric patients and geriatric medicine in Ireland. She found that generally physiotherapists had a positive attitude towards

2

old people, finding them interesting, cheerful, wise and capable of adjusting to change. The attitudes towards the old person as a patient were less clear. They agreed that the older person presented a challenge in rehabilitation, but they showed a reluctance to take up this challenge. Only 3.4 per cent considered geriatric physiotherapy as a first choice of career. The findings may indicate that the physiotherapist's professional training has not equipped her sufficiently to accept that her role in the treatment and care of patients does not lie exclusively within the realms of immediate healing. This is supported by the findings of Wagstaff, Jackson and Wheeler (1985) in a study of student physiotherapists and practitioners in which they found curing gave pre-eminence to caring. Clinical experience in geriatric hospitals while training was perceived, both by those who had previous clinical experience and by those who had not, to be of great value for increasing knowledge and understanding of the problems of the older patient.

BIOLOGICAL ASPECTS OF AGEING

People with the same chronological age may have different biological ages. Some people appear to age more rapidly than others. Everyone will know individuals in their 90s who are extremely fit and others who are in their 60s and 70s who have deteriorated significantly. Organs within the same individual age at different rates. A list of the biological changes that occur with age is rather depressing and it should be remembered that every individual does not develop all the changes. However, it is important to be aware of these changes if one is to approach the investigation and treatment of illness in this age group correctly.

Some of the age changes that occur in different systems are described in later chapters of this book. Thinning of the subcutaneous supporting tissue leads to wrinkling of the skin. The skin capillaries bleed more easily, giving rise to senile purpura. This is usually seen on the extensor surfaces of the forearms. Very mild trauma may be sufficient to produce marked bruising. Warty papillomata are commonly seen on the trunk and sometimes on the limbs and face.

There may be a slow progressive loss of hearing, which is known as presbycusis. High-frequency tones are lost initially and perception becomes particularly difficult in noisy surroundings. There is also an intolerance of loud noise and it is a mistake to shout at older patients. It is much more important to speak slowly and distinctly. Apart from hearing, the ear has an important role in maintaining balance. Degenerative changes in the semi-circular canals will impair balance and predispose to falls.

About 40 per cent of old people develop a whitish opaque ring around the eyes known as arcus senilis. It is due to the deposition of fatty substances. It does not cause the visual problems that most people experience as they get older. With increasing age, the ability of the lens to focus at different distances is impaired and it is because of this phenomenon, known as presbyopia, that most older people require glasses for reading. Vision may also be impaired due to cataract, glaucoma or senile macular degeneration. Degenerative changes within the lens lead to cataract formation with opacification and increased rigidity of the lens. Senile cataract formation is almost always bilateral. Interference with the aqueous drainage of the eye leads to increased pressure within the eyeball, a condition known as glaucoma. Glaucoma is found in about 3 per cent of people over the age of 50. Ischaemic changes in the retina may lead to degenerative changes in the fundus of the eye. This is known as senile macular degeneration. Vision is gradually impaired and eventually it may be virtually lost. Both cataract and glaucoma are amenable to surgery. However, the results of cataract surgery may be disappointing if there is underlying retinal degeneration, or if the patient is confused. Poor eyesight is frequently overlooked as a cause of immobility in old age. The physiotherapist should always assess the patient's ability to distinguish objects in his immediate environment.

Liver and kidney changes with age are particularly important in relation to drug treatment (see Chapter 12). Muscle power diminishes in those who do not exercise regularly and in advanced old age, bones become thinner (osteoporosis) and this predisposes to fractures (see Chapter 6). Reserve cardiac and respiratory function are diminished and this may become significant when the patient is stressed during an illness. In a similar way, reduced mental reserve predisposes to acute confusional states. Several changes have been described in the neurons of the ageing brain such as the deposition of lipofusein pigment and loss of mitochondria within the cells. These changes may lead to a diminished mental agility and impaired memory and learning ability. The mechanism controlling posture, anti-gravity support, balance and moving equipoise may also be affected (Adams 1977). Visual spatial perception and discrimination may be less accurate because of degenerative changes in the occipital lobe of the brain. Degenerative changes in the nervous system may also involve the temperature-regulating mechanism and predispose to hypothermia.

SOCIAL ASPECTS OF AGEING

The social standing of older people within society reflects the political and economic structure of that society as well as the cultural values, beliefs and divisions. Improved social policies in developed countries have occurred as a result of more compassionate attitudes. Old age is rarely a period of social or economic expansion for the individual and indeed, the limitations in lifestyle imposed on people who were reasonably affluent in their younger years may lead to a feeling of being relatively underprivileged (Coni, Davison and Webster 1977). Many older people who have been hovering on the poverty line for most of their lives will feel genuinely deprived in old age. They are no longer able to cope and they usually lack the necessary knowledge to obtain their entitlements.

Deprivation can lead to nutritional problems as discussed later in this chapter. It can also lead to other problems such as hypothermia, loss of mobility, sphincter disturbances, accidents, susceptibility to illness and resistance to discharge from hospital (Coni, Davison and Webster 1977). For instance, in severely cold weather an old person with inadequate heating facilities may stay in bed. The consequence is that he is a candidate for all the complications of prolonged bed rest such as pulmonary emboli, contractures and pressure sores. If the toilet is outside, he will not empty his bowels regularly and this may lead to faecal impaction and problems with bladder and rectal control. Similarly, economy in electricity bills may lead to inadequate lighting and falls may occur as a consequence.

Social isolation and desolation are two great problems for the elderly. Social isolation may stem from death of relatives or from poor family relationships. In modern society, children often move long distances from their parents and thus are unable to support them as in the extended-family system of the past. Retirement can be a source of social isolation as it suddenly cuts people off from friendships and associations at work. There is a growing awareness of the importance of preparing adequately for retirement and an increasing number of firms are organising pre-retirement courses for their staff. One of the functions of these pre-retirement courses is the dissemination of knowledge about health in old age. The physiotherapist with experience of the problems of older people should participate in such courses.

Physical disability is a major cause of social isolation. Often gradually increasing immobility is attributed to 'old age'. However, immobility in old age should be looked upon in the same way as one would regard a high temperature in younger patients — it tells us that there is something wrong (see Chapter 3, p. 22).

Desolation stems from the death of a spouse or some other close relative or friend. This can have very marked consequences in old age. The individual may become depressed and very apathetic. The incidence of suicide is increased after bereavement. There is also an increased susceptibility to physical illness and this results in considerably higher mortality amongst the survivors of bereavement.

Social isolation and frailty make the elderly an easy prey for thieves and vandals. The invasion of their privacy has major consequences for the older person and a seemingly minor theft can lead to a whole range of complications such as depression, physical illness, immobility and even death (Coakley and Woodford-Williams 1979).

NUTRITION

Undernutrition in childhood and early adult life is less common in western countries today, when compared with the situation earlier in the century. In fact, the pendulum would appear to have swung in the opposite direction and scientists are now studying the effects of overfeeding in these age groups. Despite the virtual elimination of undernutrition in younger people, it remains a serious problem in the older age groups. It is usually a result of a combination of social factors and disease.

Many old people are socially isolated and they may become apathetic about their own welfare. They may also be ignorant of the requirements of a balanced diet and poverty may restrict their choice of food. Physical and mental disability can impair their ability to obtain and to prepare food for consumption. Mastication may be a problem with badly fitting dentures. Impaired absorption in the bowel may also contribute to deficiency states, particularly affecting folic acid, vitamin B_{12}, fat-soluble vitamins and fat. Undernutrition can give rise to considerable disability in old age. Iron, vitamin B_{12} and folate deficiency can all lead to neurological disability. Scurvy, the infamous affliction of sailors years ago, is still seen occasionally, especially in elderly men. Low levels of vitamin C in the blood have been reported in institutionalised old people and in old people receiving meals-on-wheels. These findings have been attributed to the destruction of the vitamin C content during cooking, the delay in delivery of the meal and an inadequate supply of fresh fruit (Exton-Smith and Overstall 1979). Wound-healing may be delayed in patients with vitamin C deficiency and the administration of vitamin C may accelerate the healing of pressure sores by increasing the formation of collagen. Vitamin D and calcium deficiency lead to bone and muscle diseases and these can have a profound effect on an old person's mobility. This problem is discussed in detail in Chapter 6 (p. 93).

Disability consequent on malnutrition can be prevented. There must be a greater public awareness of the problem and health workers in the community should be constantly on the alert for elderly patients who might be malnourished. The housebound elderly, particularly those living alone, are most at risk.

UNREPORTED ILLNESS

Old people often feel unwell, have pain and may experience difficulty in leading an ordinary life. They and their relatives frequently do not report this to their doctors. In a pioneering study in 1964, Williamson and his colleagues found that in a survey of elderly people living at home, almost half of the disability that was identified was unknown to the patients' doctors. Musculoskeletal problems, pain in the feet, disorders of the urinary tract, dementia and anaemia were commonly not reported to general practitioners. Several other studies have confirmed that there is a vast amount of untreated illness in elderly people living at home and this has led to increased emphasis on the importance of screening clinics. Medical treatment and rehabilitation at an early stage may prevent further deterioration and dependence (Walsh 1980).

REFERENCES

Adams, G. (1977) *Essentials of geriatric medicine*. Oxford University Press, Oxford

Coakley, D. and Woodford-Williams, E. (1979) 'The effects of burglary and vandalism on the health of old people.' *Lancet, ii*, 1066–7

Coni, N., Davison, W. and Webster, S. (1977) *Lecture Notes on Geriatrics*. Blackwell Scientific Publications, Oxford

Exton-Smith, A.N. and Overstall, P. (1979) *Geriatrics*. MTP Press, Lancaster

Finn, A.M. (1986) 'Attitudes of physiotherapists towards geriatric care.' *Physiotherapy, 72*, 3, 129–31

McTavish, D. (1971) 'Perceptions of old people.' *Gerontologist, II*, 90–101

Mills, J. (1972) 'Attitudes of undergraduate students concerning geriatric patients.' *Am. J. Occ. Ther., 26*, 4, 200–3

National Academy of Sciences (1978) 'Ageing and medical education.' *Report of a Study by a Committee of the Institute of Medicine*, Washington

Paillat, P. (1981) 'Demography.' In J. Kinnaird, J. Brotherston and J. Williamson, (eds) *The provision of care for the elderly*, Churchill Livingstone, London and New York

Peach, H. (1978) 'Career plans of student physical therapists regarding geriatric medicine.' *Age and Ageing, 7*, 57–61

Rowlings, C. (1981) *Social work with the elderly*. Allen and Unwin, London

Wagstaff, P.S., Jackson, J.A. and Wheeler, T. (1985) 'Physiotherapy — Profession, Occupation or Job?' *Physiotherapy Ireland, 6*, 2, 3–5

Walsh, B. (1980) 'Previously unrecognised treatable illness in an Irish elderly population.' *J. Irish Med. Assoc. 73*, 2, 62–7

2

General Principles

Illness and disability in the older patient are often secondary to the accumulative effects of different disease processes in several organs of the body. In contrast, sick younger patients usually have symptoms and signs that can be explained by one disease process.

MULTIPLE PATHOLOGY

The occurrence of multiple pathology is particularly common in patients over the age of 75. Often there are other elements involved such as malnutrition and social problems. The multifactorial nature of disability in the elderly should not be a cause for pessimism as frequently, much can be done to improve the situation of such patients. It is important that all the patient's problems should be identified and listed. Each problem should be investigated and the appropriate treatment should be organised. Because of the differing nature of the many problems involved, no single professional has all the answers and so a team approach is necessary. Failure to adopt a multidisciplinary problem-oriented approach could lead to serious misjudgements in treatment. For instance, there may be little point in giving physiotherapy to an immobile patient whilst ignoring the patient's dense cataracts — the latter may be the main cause of the immobility.

ATYPICAL PRESENTATION

There is often a fundamental difference in the presentation of the same disease process in younger and in older patients. These differences may be due to the altered physiology of old age (see Chapter 1). An older patient may have a life-threatening pneumonia and yet not have an elevated temperature. Myocardial infarction may present without the chest pain that is a hallmark of the condition in the young. An elderly patient may walk into casualty after a fall and yet an x-ray may reveal a fractured femoral neck (see Chapter 6). A similar fracture would cause agonising pain in a younger person.

The onset of illness is often insidious in an older person and it may be attributed to ageing. In general, the recovery from illness also takes longer than in younger patients. One of the regrettable features of certain modern hospitals is that they expect sick older people to behave like sick younger people. It is unfortunate that the efficiency of a hospital tends to be judged by the average length of patient stay and patient turnover or 'through put' rates. Early and precipitant discharge of recuperating older patients will lead to deterioration and almost inevitable readmission. There is an optimum time of discharge for each patient and all professionals treating the patient should be involved in the decision.

TEAMWORK

There is general agreement that all the professions should work closely together in caring for the elderly. It is the physiotherapist's role, along with other members of the health care team, to attempt to restore lost function, or to teach a patient to function with a given disability; to obtain maximum possible independence or minimal possible dependence. Teamwork with the patient is needed to achieve the goal of returning the disabled older patient to the community with increased independence and improved quality of life.

The team and the relative significance of each member of the team varies according to the patient's condition and according to the tasks required. Relative inputs may be perceived differently by different members of the team. 'Teamwork' is a popular term at the present time and Leeming (1982) suggests that it is an over-simplification. He says that it is more useful to consider those who need to work together in each case and that 'working together' is a more accurate description of the process than 'teamwork'.

When staff from a number of different disciplines work together, there is a real danger of misunderstandings occurring, which lead to loss of efficiency. No team can work together satisfactorily if there are constant changes in personnel brought about by a 'rotating' system of staffing. It is imperative that strong elements of continuity are preserved. Inevitably, in a team situation, it has to be accepted that there will be an overlapping role; this is common between physiotherapist and nurse and physiotherapist and occupational therapist in such activities as dressing, feeding and walking. There can be no cherishing of territories. Conflict between members of a team is inevitable and providing that this is suitably channelled, it can be a source of inspiration — a means whereby important issues are neither missed nor avoided. Leeming (1982) identified two areas of conflict. The first is the more heated variety, relating to matters such as incompatible attitudes, professional status and territory; the second is straightforward honest disagreement about day-to-day judgements and decisions. Often both kinds of conflict occur at the same time.

As in a sporting activity, a rehabilitation team needs not so much a captain as a leader and this leader is usually the consultant geriatrician. Kane (1975) defined leadership as 'any conscious act of influence over the behaviour of others'. Leeming (1982) suggests the following qualities for leadership:

1. A liking for people and an understanding of the way they behave in groups, both as individuals and as members of a profession.
2. A knowledge of the aims of the department.
3. A willingness to listen and welcome criticism.
4. A strong sense of purpose and an ability to communicate this to others.
5. A sense of humour.
6. The ability to attend meetings regularly.
7. A sense of time.

Communication with a team

If the team is to be effective, then there must be good communication between all members. Hospitals suffer from hierarchical structures and too much management at a time when modern industry is moving away from such structures. The hierarchical structures in the latter are being broken down as they are seen to be counter-productive. Good communication has to exist between all members of a team if there is to be effective action. Communication can happen in a variety of ways and in a variety of situations. It is by talking to members of the team within a department that attitudes develop. This is very important when new, junior members of staff join the team. If a department reflects enthusiasm for all the good things about being old, then a general enthusiasm will prevail, but if the attitude is one of taking part in a losing battle against physical and mental decay, then a general despondency and a feeling of uselessness will prevail. Millard (1976) comments that a service should not be geared to perceived ideas and attitudes, but should be tailored to the needs of individual patients.

If the team is to operate satisfactorily there needs to be an excellence of co-ordination of activity. Staff need to be free to get on with their own activity, but not at the expense of other members of the team. Co-ordination will occur through meetings, both formal and chance. The danger of everyone attending endless case conferences, ward rounds, the firm meeting, educational meetings and so on, is that the work pattern is destroyed and administration and management take over from care and action.

It is axiomatic for effective rehabilitation that there is the closest collaboration between the therapists and nurses to provide a consistent programme in the activities of daily life. If this does not take place, advances made in the therapy departments will be undone in the wards (Woodford-Williams 1982).

Communication, whether on a one-to-one, face-to-face basis, on a round, at a conference or via a memorandum or phone call, is hard work, requires time to organise and needs conscious effort on the part of all concerned. At any meeting it is essential that all members know in advance what is to be discussed; this necessitates an agenda that is adhered to. We have all spent and wasted time at meetings only to find relevant personnel not present. Written communication is impersonal and so requires more time spent in preparing the material. Communication does not imply simply the giving of information, but also the receiving, either through the careful reading of what others put on paper or the careful listening to verbal information.

The relatives

A progressive team will look upon the patient and the relatives as important members of the team. Relatives should be encouraged to become involved in the patient's rehabilitation programme from the very beginning. They should be made aware of the progress made. If the patient is only seen by the bedside during visiting hours, relatives may form a totally inaccurate estimate of his or her abilities. Involvement in the therapy departments will prepare a relative for assuming eventual care of the patient at home. It must be remembered that in hospital, a patient will have the doctor, nurse, physiotherapist, occupational therapist, speech therapist, etc. to take care of him. On discharge, a relative may be expected to assume part of the role of all these individual professionals in the home setting. Adequate involvement with the therapists is therefore essential. It allows relatives to discuss fears, anxieties and reservations and to gain confidence gradually. The therapist *must* make time to listen to relatives and of course, even more importantly, to the patient.

The patient

Each patient must be treated as an individual. They each have their own loves, fears and anxieties and so it is essential that the therapist should learn to listen. The patient may be very lonely and a sympathetic ear can have its own therapeutic effect. It may also be an educational experience for a young therapist. Many elderly patients have had extremely interesting lives and they often have fascinating stories to narrate. The patient must always be treated with dignity. Physiotherapists have a very personal relationship with their patients, more so than in any other discipline. Being on first-name terms may help this relationship but this should not be assumed unless the therapist is encouraged to do so by the patient. It is obviously insulting to refer to an older patient as 'pop' or 'pet' or other such terms of familiarity. The patient's sense of privacy and modesty must always be protected by the appropriate use of screens or curtains whenever necessary.

When the patient is over the acute phase of the illness, he should be encouraged to dress in his own clothes. This enhances dignity and self-respect and it also promotes a positive attitude towards rehabilitation. Finally, the therapist should encourage the patient and be enthusiastic, particularly if there is any response, no matter how small, to a particular treatment.

A THERAPEUTIC MILIEU

Failure to treat the elderly patient as an individual may result in rapid institutionalisation. The patient becomes very submissive and dependent upon 'the system'. The patient's talents and intellectual ability gradually atrophy because of lack of stimulation. Apathy replaces initiative to such an extent, that the patient becomes depersonalised and withdraws into a world of his own. Eventually the patient becomes physically dependent and incontinent. Once institutionalised it is extremely difficult to rehabilitate such a patient.

If patients are to make progress and maintain or regain their self-respect, it is essential that the emotional tone around them should be one of respect, enjoyment and a belief in their eventual recovery. Such a positive therapeutic atmosphere can only be achieved when the different professional groups in a team identify it as one of their priorities. The physiotherapist can play a very important role in developing the rehabilitation team into a 'therapeutic community'. She should also strive to improve the physical milieu and endeavour to develop an environment conducive to rehabilitation. The importance of structuring such an environment cannot be overemphasised. Efforts expended in this direction will be rewarded by better rehabilitation results and consequently, with greater job satisfaction for the therapist and greater independence for the patient.

REFERENCES

Kane, R.A. (1975) 'The interprofessional team as a small group.' *Social Work in Health Care I*

Leeming, J.T. (1982) 'Attitudes, teamwork, co-ordination and communication.' In D. Coakley, (ed). *Establishing a geriatric service*, Croom Helm, London

Millard, P.H. (1976) 'Attitudes and geriatrics.' In J.T. Leeming, (ed). *Doctors and old age, British Geriatrics Society*, Mitcham

Woodford-Williams, E. (1982) 'The efficiency and quality of the service.' In D. Coakley, (ed). *Establishing a geriatric service*, Croom Helm, London

3

Physiotherapy Assessment

When thinking of assessment in terms of the elderly, it is important to appreciate that people are not ill and in need of care just because they are old. Assessment of the elderly is often complicated by the presence of multiple pathology as pointed out in Chapter 2. There is the possible co-existence of physical, psychological, nutritional and social disturbance in the same individual. In the older patient, the assessment is made more complex in that the manifestations of a disease are often different from those in younger people, indeed often expected symptoms seem lacking (see Chapter 2). Such difficulties emphasise the need for more accurate and complete assessment in an older patient, not a scant summary of mobility.

PATIENT HISTORY

Assessment of an elderly patient may require more time and more patience than with a younger patient. More time is needed because of the possibility of impaired sight and hearing, impairment of memory and confusion. It is a pointless exercise to shout at deaf people; it merely accentuates vowels and obscures consonants. Questions need to be simple and straightforward and frequently it will be necessary to take a history from some other person, ideally a close relative or the person most closely associated with the patient. Tact is required in acquiring information in this way. It is not always easy to interpret symptoms: for example, it does not necessarily follow that an inability to walk is due to a disturbance of the locomotor system. It is important to find out how long symptoms have been present and the sequence in which symptoms have appeared. From the physiotherapist's point of view, the family history is needed in order to evaluate what might be expected from the patient's relatives in terms of care.

THE HOME ENVIRONMENT

It is essential to find out about the site of and the number of stairs, the lavatory, bathing facilities, the water supply, cooking arrangements, heating, lighting and likely accident hazards. A home visit may be necessary to obtain accurate information and this may be carried out with other members of the team such as the occupational therapist or the medical social worker (see Chapter 14). It is not so much the essential of good as opposed to bad housing, more an assessment of appropriate as opposed to inappropriate housing. If a patient is unlikely ever to cope with stairs, a house in which a flight of stairs has to be negotiated may be deemed inappropriate. A patient may be thought to be permanently incontinent by a family or worse still by medical colleagues, when the problem is that of lack of mobility or inappropriate toilet facilities. The size of the lavatory is crucial if walking aids or wheelchairs are to be considered.

Inadequate cooking facilities may result in a patient suffering from nutritional disorders. Any form of adequate heating today is expensive. The choice may have to be between being cold or being hungry. Most accidents happen in the home and are more likely to involve elderly people. By far the most common cause of fatal home accidents is a fall. Accidental falls occur on stairs where there is no hand rail. Loose rugs, slippery and wet floors, inappropriate footwear and old furniture are all possible hazards (see Chapter 6, p. 108). Questions need to be asked about who looks after the home and who looks after the patient. Independence is to be favoured, but if a highly independent old person is suddenly rendered immobile, a crisis rapidly develops, whereas if a degree of dependence already exists, the crisis may not be so acute or grave. It is of fundamental importance to assess the support given by family and friends. It has to be accepted that even the strongest bonds of affection may be damaged or destroyed by difficulties that arise from illness.

GENERAL ASSESSMENT

As with all patients, first impressions can be very helpful. With elderly patients, factors such as alertness and general demeanour provide important information about their mental state. There may be signs of neglect, which may be self-neglect or neglect on the part of relatives.

In terms of general observation, the skin is an important tissue to assess. Bruises may indicate recent falls. The state of pressure areas should be noted, as prompt treatment is required at the earliest evidence of a sore.

During all assessment procedures, the physiotherapist should consider the functional implications of abnormality. Cowdrey (1976) has stated that to manage independently, a patient should be able to walk or transfer from a bed to a chair without being lifted, have normal, or nearly normal control of excretory function, be able to take care of personal needs such as eating, dressing and bathing, and possess a reasonable mental state. Bruell and Peszcynski (1958) consider that the ability to move about on one's own is a prerequisite to independence.

SPECIFIC ASSESSMENT PROCEDURES

Respiratory system

An estimate of cough and sputum produced each day is of relevance: although many old people will deny the presence of a cough, they will discuss happily the quantity and quality of phlegm that is produced. Some old people without a respiratory disorder will complain of breathlessness on climbing stairs or hurrying. However, an assessment of distance managed on flat ground and the presence or absence of breathlessness during dressing is of value.

The strength of a cough is important, as a weak cough is likely to present the physiotherapist with greater problems if a chest infection is present. The quality of the sputum should be investigated; mucoid sputum implies no severe current infection. An increased respiratory rate may be the first indication of a pneumonic process in the elderly. Prolonged expiration through pursed lips and rapid inspiration is characteristic of obstruction of the airways. Most patients are well able to cope with ventilatory tests using the Vitalograph and Wright's Peak Flow Meter.

17

Nervous system

Assessment of the nervous system of the elderly patient is quite different to that of other age groups. Certain abnormalities are in a way 'normal' or at least of little significance. Ankle jerks, for example, are commonly absent. Sensation can be difficult to assess because of communication difficulties. Elderly people may talk of 'dizziness' and 'fainting'. In order to extract more precise information, it is necessary to find out what brought on the 'dizziness', how long it lasted and whether there was true loss of consciousness. For instance, if the 'dizziness' is felt when the patient gets out of bed in the morning, it may be that the symptom is brought about by a transient drop in blood pressure.

It is important to assess the patient for any evidence of mental impairment. Simple psychometric tests may be used to assess intellectual capacity. Recent and remote memory, orientation for time, place and person and the ability to carry out simple calculations should all be tested. The therapist should also be on the alert for signs of depression. Depression or intellectual impairment may frustrate rehabilitation attempts, even more so if they are missed on initial assessment. The importance of asking about falls and instability is stressed in Chapter 6.

Head and neck

Passive neck movements should be tested. Limitation of movement is common in cervical spondylosis, especially lateral flexion, whereas rigidity of the neck in all planes occurs in Parkinson's disease and in patients with bilateral pyramidal tract disorders.

Visual fields should be tested, as diminution will have an effect on function and balance. Loss of vertical- and horizontal-space perception is a common problem in hemiplegics and such sensory perceptual evaluation helps to explain the difficulty these patients find in assuming the upright posture and affords a better appreciation of ensuing gait problems.

The face should be assessed to determine asymmetry or weakness. Facial movement should be looked at on voluntary effort and this is often the best method to determine symmetry and asymmetry. Weakness of upper facial musculature leads to loss of transverse brow creases.

Speech should be listened to carefully. First it is necessary to distinguish between disorders of phonation and articulation, when speech seems soft and slurred, and disorders of dysphasia. When a patient has not got teeth in place, speech may be affected. Movements of the tongue and position of the tongue are relevant in the manner in which they will affect speech. Try speaking normally with a retracted tongue and you will appreciate the difficulty that some hemiplegic patients find in communicating clearly. Hearing should also be tested, with particular emphasis on the hearing field.

One needs to establish whether the patient is left-handed or right-handed. It should be remembered that in the elderly age group, there will be left-handed 'naturals' who were 'converted' at school.

Upper limb

Pain and stiffness in the upper limb are two important symptoms to the physiotherapist. These symptoms are common in the fingers in rheumatoid arthritis. Severe shoulder pain, especially at night, combined with gross limitation of movement (particularly lateral rotation and abduction) is typical of adhesive capsulitis (frozen shoulder). Severe bilateral pain in the shoulders without limitation of movement is typical of polymyalgia rheumatica. As a general guide for physiotherapists during assessment, pain in the upper limb resulting from joint disease is usually accompanied by limitation of movement and pain from other causes, including referred pain, will not be so accompanied. Disorders may give rise to loss of function without pain. Loss of function of gradual onset (as for example joint disease, Parkinson's disease) should be distinguished from those of sudden onset (e.g. CVA or fracture). Physiotherapists should be aware of the overall pattern of involvement. An elderly person's hands tend to rest in mild ulnar deviation, which in itself is insignificant. A minor degree of thickening of the palmar fascia is very common, being seen in 10 per cent of elderly men (Caird and Judge 1976). Dupuytren's contracture is not uncommon.

The range of movement in elderly people is very similar to that of young people; limitation of joint movement is not a feature of getting old. Minor degrees of limitation may occur after certain pathologies, but may be quite asymptomatic and cause no loss of function and are therefore unimportant. As joints are being assessed for range of movement, muscle tone may be tested. Parkinson's rigidity is most easily detected at the wrist and elbow. Muscle tenderness may be determined by squeezing the muscles of the forearms and upper arm gently.

Outstretched hands are assessed for tremor or drifting of a limb. As with patients of all age groups, comparison is made between both sides when assessing muscle power. Reflexes should also be compared and sensation should be tested. It is important to test joint-position, particularly in the hemiplegic patient who may show signs of neglect or denial of a limb. This, if demonstrated, creates problems in rehabilitation as the limb may not be used despite good return of power and all stimuli may be ignored.

Lower limb

The main symptoms associated with the lower limb are pain, gait disturbances, weakness and swelling. Sudden onset of pain in the hip and thigh may be due to fracture or acute arthritis. Slowly developing pain is probably due to osteoarthrosis. Painful knees are extremely common in the elderly. Pain and stiffness in the calf occurring on exercise is characteristic of arterial disease (patients will often refer to the pain as 'cramp'). This is not to be confused with cramp in the legs at night which is quite common and for which there is no obvious cause. Pain in the feet is not uncommon. Chiropody problems must be looked for and referral to the chiropodist is essential. Such problems, even though they can have a profound effect on mobility, are commonly overlooked. Difficulty in walking may be due to pain or due to neurological abnormality.

Assessment should include: details of distance, effects of stopping, difficulty in getting out of a chair, difficulty on stairs, ramps and slopes and difficulties experienced on different floor coverings and varying surfaces. Assessment of the lower limb is carried out as described previously for the upper limb. It is important to note the state of the skin for care in handling during treatment and for evidence of recent bruising, indicating the possibility of a fall. Pulses should be palpated.

Back

It is important that the physiotherapist should remember that there are many causes of back pain, some due to mechanical derangement, which may be treated, some with no relevance to the physiotherapist and some, for example, due to metastatic deposits which contraindicate certain or all physiotherapy treatments. The purpose of assessment is therefore in part to identify the basic cause of pain. If a patient has complained of pain over many years, then the cause is unlikely to be sinister. Pain of recent onset or pain after a fall may be due to a fracture or metastatic deposit. Severe, persistent pain in the lumbo-dorsal region unaffected by movement or coughing and present all the time, may indicate pancreatic carcinoma.

Gait

If fit enough and able, a patient's walking should be observed. Shoes should be worn and not slippers. Not only is gait itself of relevance, but careful note should be made of associated movements in the arm and trunk. From a functional point of view, it is essential to assess the safety of gait and the manner in which aids are used.

Balance

In an assessment of the patient's balance, it is necessary to answer two main questions:

1. What does a patient need to do?
2. What is their ability to do it?

In each of the fundamental starting positions, three main elements are assessed. The following is an example of assessment in the seated position:

1. What support is required to maintain balance over a base?

   (a) Can the patient sit unassisted with both feet on the floor with no support to the back or arms?
   (b) For how long?
   (c) How much support is required?
   (d) Is extra support required when the patient's eyes are closed?

2. What is the patient's response to external forces tending to disturb him?

    (a) Response of arms.
    (b) Attempt at correction.
    (c) Ability to establish a new stable position.

3. What degree of independent activity may be carried out?

    (a) Can the patient retain balance while moving his head?
    (b) Can the patient retain balance while moving his trunk?
    (c) Can the patient retain balance while moving his arms and trunk?

The same plan for assessment of balance may be chosen for any of the fundamental starting positions. If, for example, a patient can achieve 3(c) in the standing position, then he will be ready to walk independently.

Muscle strength

Methods of grading muscle strength and power have been developed over many years. According to de Vries (1970), no set values have been developed to establish an accurate basis for interpreting normal strength in the elderly. The standard format for measuring muscle power is a six-point scale known as the 'Oxford Scale'. However, Ransome (1980) suggested a three-point scale as being adequate for assessing the older patient:

    3. Poor (nil or slight strength).
    2. Fair (token resistance permitted).
    1. Good (token resistance permitted).

It is not strength *per se*, that is relevant, but to what extent a degree of strength is required in order to permit a satisfactory level of physical function.

Mobility

It is the combination of mobility, strength and balance that determine the functional capability of the patient. The School of Physiotherapy at the University of Dublin uses an assessment chart (Fig. 3.1) designed by Ann Finn, a staff member. This incorporates several

Figure 3.1: Basic assessment of mobility

Surname: ....   Admitted ....
Forenames: ....   Diagnosis ....
Address ....

PHYSICAL	PSYCHOLOGICAL	SOCIAL
Can the patient walk	☐ Orientated	☐ Marital status
☐ Independently	☐ Disorientated	☐ i.e. Single/Married/Widow(er)
☐ With an aid	☐ Apathetic	☐ Living alone
☐ With support of 2 people	☐ Depressed	☐ Living with relatives
☐ Unable to walk	**Motivation**	☐ House
	☐ Good	☐ Flat
Type of gait	☐ Poor	☐ Stairs
☐ Ataxic type	**Comprehension**	
☐ Shuffling type	☐ Co-operative	**Occupation**
☐ Slow	☐ Non co-operative	☐ Retired
☐ Spastic	**Type of aid used**	Hobbies/Interests
☐ Festinating	☐ Stick	
	☐ Tripod	
Cause of Dependency	☐ Quadrupod	Other medical problems
☐ Imbalance	☐ Walking frame	
☐ Joint immobility	☐ Rollator	
☐ Deformity	☐ Crutches	
☐ Muscle weakness	**A. Main problems encountered**	
☐ Fear of falling		
☐ Pain		
☐ Trauma		
☐ Impaired vision		
☐ Impaired hearing		
☐ Impaired speech		
☐ Respiratory dysfunction	**B. Main objective**	
☐ Dyspnoea on exertion		
☐ Continent		
☐ Incontinent		
☐ Pressure sores		
☐ Pressure ulcers		
☐ Upper limit rt/lt	**C. Further comments**	
☐ Weakness		
☐ Tremor		
☐ Joint immobility		
☐ Postural deformity		

Source: School of Physiotherapy, Dublin

aspects of mobility and functional capability. The patient is graded after Ransome (1980) in relation to both mobility and capability:

3. Good (full or nearly full mobility).
2. Fair (limited mobility but allows reasonable function).
1. Poor (limited mobility — function impossible).

3. Good (manages alone).
2. Fair (manages with supervision).
1. Poor (manages with physical help).

Frazer (1979) devised an eight-point scale that is related to function and not to disability or pathological condition. In this way, it allows for changes in functional ability, which may be achieved with treatment, but which are unrelated to changes in physical condition:

1. No disability.
2. Independently mobile.
3. Limited mobility.
4. Housebound — able to do light housework.
5. Housebound — limited to self-care activities.
6. Housebound — requiring help with self-care activities.
7. Chairbound — requiring help with self-care activities.
8. Totally dependent.

The physiotherapist and occupational therapist should work closely together in the functional assessment of patients and their ability to perform activities of daily living. A series of items that are typically included in the formulation of an 'Activities of Daily Living' chart are included in Appendix 1 (p. 212).

WHEELCHAIR ASSESSMENT

It is essential that a wheelchair be correctly prescribed to meet the needs of the patient and his or her carers. It must be the type that offers the support required, is the correct size for comfort and the prevention of decubiti and has the features and accessories needed for safety and maximum independence. There are several different types:

Electric wheelchairs

An electric wheelchair is selected for those patients unable to propel a standard wheelchair. Some models are small and manoeuvrable with a moulded or cushioned seat and a centre bar and control stick. Others are similar to a standard chair with a power-drive control box located on the left or right side near the arm rest. A stick on top of the control box is held and pushed in the direction in which the patient wishes the chair to move.

Self-propelling standard wheelchairs

The common type of wheelchair has a metal frame, canvas or cloth seating and four wheels. Two of the wheels have a large diameter (about 56 cm (21 in)) and may have a separate rim for the patient to use to propel the chair. The other two wheels have a smaller diameter (about 18 cm (7 in)) and are freely pivoting castors. Most commonly, the larger wheels are at the back.

Transit or pushchairs

These chairs have four small wheels (about 30 cm (12 in)), either with two pivoted and two fixed wheels or with all four wheels fixed. They may be rigid or capable of being folded for ease of transport and storage.

Coates and King (1983) define the following criteria for wheelchair assessment:

Size of patient

Wheelchairs are designed primarily for patients of normal height and weight, which may present problems for the very large patient. Patients weighing over 114 kg (250 lb) need heavy duty chairs; those below 102 kg (224 lb) may be prescribed a lightweight chair. Wherever possible, the lightest possible chair available should be prescribed, as chairs may weigh from 15–27 kg (33–59 lb) and the heavier the chair the less manoeuvrable it becomes.

Ability to use limbs

It is important to determine whether the patient is capable of using one or both hands and whether they have enough strength in the arms to propel the chair under normal conditions. If the chair is to be used solely indoors, the patient should be assessed for ability to propel the chair over carpet, linoleum, rugs and so on. If outdoor use is envisaged, assessment on road surfaces, inclines, curbs and steps must be made. It is important to know where the patient is going to use the chair. If the chair is to be used primarily indoors, then the chair will need to be light, narrow and manoeuvrable. If it is to be used primarily outdoors it will need to be robust, with large wheels and pneumatic tyres. Chairs should be comfortable as well as providing optimum mobility. If a patient is not capable of performing these functions in the appropriate environment, the decision may be taken to provide a powered chair. The functional effectiveness of the limbs in propelling a wheelchair is dependent on both muscle power and range of movement in the joints. If a patient is unable to either self-propel or work the controls of a powered unit, the latter either from physical inability or temperament, a simple transit chair should be considered.

Vision

Self-propelled wheelchairs may be potentially hazardous for patients with limited vision. However, it is unwise to determine a fixed level of visual disability where a patient should not be prescribed a self-propelled wheelchair because of the ability of certain patients to adapt to their visual limitations.

Neurological deficits

Some patients, although possessing the necessary range of joint movement and muscle strength to self-propel a wheelchair, may be so lacking in sensory appreciation as to make the necessary physical responses impossible.

Mental capabilities

Certain patients are emotionally and temperamentally incapable of operating any form of wheelchair and, for them, operator-controlled chairs are the only solution.

General health

Patients with severe cardiac or respiratory disease, although capable of operating manually propelled wheelchairs, may have to be dissuaded from such a procedure because of the effects of physical exertion on the underlying pathology.

It is also important that the capabilities of a carer or operator of a transit chair are assessed. It may be that certain elderly partners will not have the necessary capabilities or may themselves be put at risk through the effort required.

There are a number of accessories available for chairs that should be considered — back rests to give adequate support to the back and possibly support for the head, arm rests which may or may not be removable and shaped so that they fit under tables, seat cushions, foot rests, different-sized wheels and wheel attachments such as capstans, leg rests and also variable positions and locations for hand-brakes.

REFERENCES

Bruell, J.H. and Peszcynski, M. (1958) 'Perceptions of verticality: hemiplegic patients in relation to rehabilitation.' *Clin. Orthop. 12*, 124–9

Caird, F.I. and Judge, T.G. (1976) *Assessment of the elderly patient.* Pitman Medical, London

Coates, H. and King, A. (1983) *The patient assessment — a handbook for therapists.* Churchill Livingstone, Edinburgh

Cowdrey, P.V. (1976) *The care of the geriatric patient.* C.V. Mosby, St Louis and London

de Vries, H. (1970) 'Physiological effect of an exercise programme upon men aged 52–88 years.' *J. Gerontol. 25*, 325–9

Frazer, F.W. (1979) 'Assessment of elderly patients.' *Physiotherapy 65,7*, 212–3

Ransome, H.E. (1980) 'Role of the physiotherapist in homes for the elderly.' *Physiotherapy, 66,10*, 324–31

4

Neurological Disability

There appears to be a moderate fall in the weight and size of the brain with advancing age. This is evident from postmortem studies and studies using axial tomography (CT scans). The fact that nerve cells cannot reproduce may be an important factor in the changes observed in the nervous system. Beginning at the age of 20, there is a gradual loss of neurons in particular areas of the brain. There are also internal and external structural changes in ageing nerve-cell bodies (Brody 1982). For instance, loss of dendritic processes and synaptic contacts have been observed and it has been postulated that there is an increase in the number of shrinking and dying cells as the brain ages (Bowen and Davison 1982).

Peripheral nerves also show some degenerative changes with age. Thinning of the myelin sheaths has been observed. These changes lead to a slowing of conduction velocity and diminution or loss of certain reflexes, particularly the ankle jerk. Vibration sense also diminishes with age. Proprioceptive feedback also declines and this may be related to age changes in the neurons of the dorsal column. Although subjective sensory changes such as parasthesia are common, the pain threshold is increased in old age.

Ageing is associated with a decrease in strength, speed and co-ordination. The decrease in strength may be related to the decrease in size of motor units (Gutman and Hanzlikova 1966). There is also a decrease in the diameter of muscle fibres (Rowe 1969). Campbell and McComas (1973) have demonstrated a loss of the number of functioning motor units in old age. In addition to peripheral mechanisms such as these, it would seem logical to believe that changes in motor performance would also involve changes in central mechanisms.

MOBILITY

Elderly people will develop contractures readily and quickly if they are bedridden for a time, or spend the greater part of the day in a chair, or are immobilised in a cast of some type. Immobilisation of the whole of the body or of a part of the body should be for as short a period as possible. As with any group of patients, it is essential to know or evaluate the cause of the limitation in movement. For instance, there may be pain that induces muscle spasm and thereby limits movement. A suitable treatment would, in this instance, be relief of pain. Coakley and Snell (1979) drew attention to the importance of unrecognised fractures in old age as a cause of immobility. Many drugs may cause immobility, inducing oversedation, postural hypotension or parkinsonism. Depression should never be forgotten and it is easily missed in an older patient. Chiropody may make a tremendous difference to an immobile older patient who has painful feet.

During acute illness, most elderly patients are immobile. However, the patient should be mobilised as early as possible. Many years ago in a famous essay, Asher (1947) highlighted the problems of prolonged bed rest. Complications include apathy, venous thrombosis, pulmonary embolism, contractures, incontinence and pressure sores.

If the cause of limitation is a developing contracture, 'passive' stretching may be performed by the therapist and 'active' stretching by the patient. Alternatively, mechanical stretching may be given by means of an 'appliance', such as a brace with a turntable or a ratchet device. When appliances are used, there is the danger of the development of pressure sores and extreme care should be taken when they are used. Contractures are one of the nightmares that a physiotherapist faces and often a feeling of helplessness ensues; too often the cause is neglect. Contractures may be avoided if the patient undergoes a full range of activity for all joints each day. Depending upon the underlying conditions, these may need to be active, active/assisted or passive. Accessory movements must not be neglected, especially in the hands and feet. It must be appreciated that contractures can occur in spite of physiotherapy. For example, a patient with brain failure may adopt the foetal position and resist all attempts at passive stretching.

PARKINSON'S DISEASE

Parkinson's disease and the parkinsonian syndrome comprise a group of disorders characterised by tremor and disturbance of voluntary movement, posture and balance. Parkinson's disease was first described by a London general practitioner in 1817. The disease affects about one per 1,000 of the total population. In persons over the age of 55 its incidence rises to about ten per 1,000, so it is the second most common neurological disorder of the elderly after 'stroke'.

Non-specific complaints such as tiredness, slowness and muscle aches, which could be prodromal symptoms of Parkinson's disease, may be attributed to old age and arthritis. It can be confused with depression because of the generalised psychomotor retardation. The combination of anxiety, excitement and awareness of being watched may all unmask a latent tremor that may present in only one of the patient's hands. If in walking, the patient exhibits normal step-length, arm-swing and turning, then it is unlikely that the patient is suffering from Parkinson's disease. However, there is a tendency to explain away certain symptoms in the elderly such as the inability to do up buttons, or to cut up meat or to sign the pension book as slowness due to arthritis.

Rigidity and bradykinesia are two essential features of Parkinson's disease. Autonomic dysfunction with posture and balance defects, bladder dysfunction and mental impairment are likely to occur in elderly people. In younger patients, the neuropathological changes are concentrated in the substantia nigra, but in older patients, changes are found in other areas of the brain. This probably accounts for the differences in clinical presentation. A resting tremor forms part of the classic triad, but its presence is not essential to make the diagnosis and it is often absent in late-onset parkinsonism.

So called senile, essential or familial tremor is frequently diagnosed as parkinsonism. However, in contrast to the tremor of Parkinson's disease, essential tremor disappears with complete relaxation. It is also the only tremor that involves the jaw, face and voice. Essential tremor has been associated with accelerated neurological ageing and with disorders of gait and balance. Patients with essential tremor are not improved by anti-Parkinson medication.

Multiple small infarcts throughout the brain due to occlusion of small blood vessels may also produce symptoms and signs similar to Parkinson's disease. Clinical features of multi-infarct disease include hypertonia, impaired facial and fine movements and a 'march-à-petit pas' type of gait. Reflexes are brisk and plantars are extensor, indicating cortico-spinal pathology. There may also be emotional lability.

In elderly patients, the physical signs of parkinsonism are similar to those in younger people and the main problems are the emotional state of the patient and an undue sensitivity to the drugs commonly used for this condition. Side-effects are common and disorientation, aggressive behaviour, ideas of persecution, depression and hallucinations may be present.

The finding that parkinsonism was related to a deficiency of dopamine (Brodie and Shore 1957) in the extrapyramidal system has transformed treatment. The level of dopamine in the brain can be raised by giving levodopa. Clinical trials began in 1961 (Cotzias, Van Woert and Schiffer 1967). Hildick-Smith (1979) has shown that a benefit period of three to seven years may be expected in those patients who respond to levodopa; after this time, there may be a deterioration with such side effects as dyskinesias, which may be due to the disease itself or the result of the accumulation of levodopa therapy. She further showed that patients with so-called benign parkinsonism show little deterioration over 15 to 20 years, whilst those with tremor alone may be better treated with physiotherapy, advice, reassurance and regular review. Progression to levodopa therapy is made when the patient develops significant disability.

Physiotherapy still has an important role in the care of the Parkinson patient. The patient must realise that physiotherapy cannot reverse any of the changes that have occurred within the central nervous system, but can minimise the effect of these changes by encouraging normal activities. For this reason, it is best that patients have periods of rest from treatment. The aims of physiotherapy are to relieve the patient's symptoms and to give the patient and relatives advice and assistance.

Treatment will focus upon means of reducing rigidity and upon assisting the patient in balance reactions. Because of damage to the basal ganglia, the patient will exhibit difficulty in initiating movement as a result of excessive postural fixation, loss of rotation and loss of rhythm, especially in walking. It will be observed that the patient adopts a fixed head and shoulder position and because of the loss or lack of the rotational component of movement, activity does not exist or the patient moves around 'as a whole'. As a consequence of rigidity and the general increase in muscle tone, there is opposition to movement so activity is produced slowly and the normal automatic postural adjustments are absent. The abnormalities in movement that exist deny the patient the normal sensory feedback, so abnormality becomes 'normality' as far as the patient is concerned.

Harrison (1982) advocates the application of cold packs prior to activity to help promote relaxation of rigidity. Proprioceptive neuromuscular facilitation techniques will assist limb and trunk activities. Emphasis should be placed initially on trunk activity and on the proximal limb joints before the intermediate and distal limb joints. Isotonic rather than isometric techniques are employed as it is dynamic activity that the patient lacks. They have an excess of static activity due to the disease process. 'Pumping-up' activity is used, which utilises rhythmical activity. Movement is first produced passively. As rigidity eases, active-assisted movements follow, then active and finally resisted movement. Similarly, the patient utilises 'pumping' activity prior to walking by marking time on the spot. The patient is encouraged to introduce arm swing and to lengthen the stride of gait. Many of these activities are similar to the type of exercise advocated by Frenkel (Wale 1961). These consist of a carefully planned series of exercises that aim at making the patient employ what is left to him of muscle sense. Commands are given in an even manner, frequently to counting. Each set of exercises must be mastered by the patient. Progression is not achieved by increasing strength, but by increasing the complexity of the activity. Exercise in full range is followed by parts of range and rest is given frequently.

As Parkinson described, patients have a tendency to adopt a fixed posture which affects the patient in many ways. It inhibits respiratory movement, makes balance reactions slower and inhibits speech, mastication and deglutination. Such posture will also cause pain. Patients should be encouraged to perform exercises and activity of the cervical spine; movements of the head should lead movement of the trunk. Thoracic mobility will aid ventilation and breathing exercises are given in an attempt to avoid the danger of chest complications which are life-threatening to such patients.

The mask-like expression of a Parkinson's patient arises because of inactivity in the facial muscles. In addition, difficulty in feeding occurs because of loss of function in the buccinator muscle so that food and drink tend to dribble from the mouth; this is embarrassing for the patient and socially unacceptable. Inactivity of the tongue produces both deglutition and speech problems. Stimulation of the tongue and facial muscles may be brought about by icing of the mouth and tongue, followed by proprioceptive neuromuscular facilitation techniques.

At a recent workshop, Kinnear (1986) emphasised the importance of the multidisciplinary team in the management of this disease as well as the need for early referral.

Aims

The aims of long-term management should be:

1. To maintain the patient at the highest level of functional independence for as long as possible on a minimal dose of anti-parkinsonian drugs;
2. To monitor the patient objectively and at regular intervals so that relevant intervention can be directed according to the changing needs;
3. To prevent or reduce mobility problems and deformities;
4. To educate the patient, relatives and care staff in the management of the disease.

General practitioners should be encouraged to refer patients for physiotherapy whenever they diagnose Parkinson's disease. On referral there should be:

1. Initial discussion;
2. Physical assessment;
3. Home assessment;
4. Treatment;
5. Advice and guidance for carers;
6. On-going care;
7. Close liaison between hospital and community staff.

Initial discussion

This may be carried out at the patient's home, in a clinic or in hospital. The patient will be encouraged to join the Parkinson's Disease Society and where possible to attend branch meetings. At this point, an explanation of Parkinson's disease may be given, together with an indication of the type of problems that may occur along with a discussion on the proposed type of treatment or management. The patient's agreement will be sought for a home assessment to be carried out and appropriate exercises will be offered.

Physical assessment

The physical assessment may be carried out using the Parkinson's disease assessment form (see pp. 36–7).

Home assessment

It is essential that the home should be assessed to ensure that the furniture and layout allow the patient to function as independently as possible. Home assessments will need to be carried out several times during a patient's illness as needs change.

Treatment

Comment has already been made on an approach to care. The overall aims may be summarised thus:

(a) To correct abnormal gait patterns;
(b) To correct or monitor poor posture;
(c) To minimise secondary muscle weakness and joint stiffness;
(d) To increase depth of respiration;
(e) To improve function;
(f) To give the patient a regime that he can carry out independently at home.

Advice and guidance for carers

As the need arises for the patients to have more assistance, the physiotherapist should be readily available to guide the carer to give assistance effectively and efficiently so that the patient will do as much as possible for himself. It should also help the carer to avoid harming her/himself in the process. In the later stages, there should be close co-operation with the community nurse. Friends and relatives must be made aware that prolonged periods of activity are to be avoided. Relatives may be shown 'pumping activity' to 'loosen' the patient. Clothes should be easy to fasten and placed to the side of the patient when dressing to encourage rotation. However, the physiotherapist should be aware that failure to achieve success with these activities can lead to the patient feeling frustrated.

On-going care

Self-referral

In the early stages, the patient may be encouraged to ring for advice on treatment when he feels the need arising. Thus a reassessment can be made to ensure that the problems can be tackled appropriately and as soon as possible.

Regular assessment

When the patient begins to require assistance the carers can request a reassessment of the situation. Preferably, regular assessments should be undertaken to ensure that problems are dealt with early, before bad habits have been allowed to develop in both patients and carers. This may avoid a crisis occurring which could necessitate a hospital admission. It may help to prevent a loss of confidence in both patient and carer and to assist in keeping the patient in his home environment for as long as possible.

Close liaison between hospital and community services

It is vitally important that there is good and effective communication between the patient, relatives, carers, hospital and community staff and services. Problems in the community should be picked up and dealt with while they are still relatively minor and not left until either the patients or their relatives cannot cope. Advice may be given on the provision of aids, such as raised seats, electric razors, toothbrushes, zips and Velcro fastenings for clothes.

Assessment

Franklyn (1986) described a form of assessment (Fig. 4.1 pp. 36–7) compiled by a Working Party of physiotherapists in conjunction

Figure 4.1: Physiotherapy assessment for idiopathic Parkinson's disease

Section One
Basic information

Patient's name ....
Address ....
....
Telephone ....
Physiotherapist ....
Referral date ....
Review date ....

Date of birth .... Sex: M/F
Age (years) ....

Referral source:	Consultant	1
	GP	2
	Other	3

Hospital (if any) ....
Hospital number ....

Social history (circle number alongside the chosen answers)

Marital status	Single	1
	Married	2
	Divorced	3
	Widowed	4

Hobbies and interests ....

Occupational	Working	1
status	Retired	2
	Housewife	3
	Other	4

Present/last paid employment ....

Accommodation (tick as necessary)
Flat (ground floor) ....
Flat (other floors) ....
Warden controlled accommodation .....
House ....
Bungalow ....
Residential care ....
Does the patient use stairs ....
lift ....
neither ....
both ....
Does the patient live alone ....

Assistance available (tick as necessary)
Household member ....
Friend/neighbour ....
Warden ....
Home help ....
District nurse ....
Meals-on-wheels ....
Social worker ....
Other (specify) ....
No assistance ....

Medical history
Age at diagnosis of PD
Years with PD
Present parkinsonian symptoms (tick as necessary)
Tremor ....
Rigidity ....
Bradykinesia ....
Speech difficulties ....
Pain ....
Freezing ....
On/off ....
Salivation ....
Swallowing difficulty ....
Other(s) (specify) ....
Pre-existing conditions limiting mobility .....
....

Medication:
a) Anti-parkinsonian ....
....
b) Other ....
....

Other relevant medical information
....
....
....
....

Section Two
Physiotherapy assessment

Beside each question on the form is a row of five boxes in which to enter the score on successive assessments
Date ....
Time of day ....
Time (hours) since last does of anti-parkinsonian drugs ....

Posture when standing: (1–4) ....
(See scoring key)

Balance

Can the patient:
1. Sit unsupported ....
2. Stand with feet together without aid ....
3. Stand on right leg (2 sec) without aid ....
4. Stand on left leg (2 sec) without aid .....

Gait

1. Initiation difficulty
Yes = 2, no = 1, unable to assess = 0 ...

2. Walking test
Distance (metres)
No. of strides ....
Time taken (sec) ....

Figure 4.1: *continued*

3. Gait description
Heel/toe = 3, flat footed = 2, toe/heel = 1,
not assessed = 0
....

4. Type of walking aid used ....

5. Arm swing

Full bi-lateral = 4, uni-lateral reduction = 3,
unilateral loss = 2, bi-lateral loss = 1,
unable to assess = 0 ....

Climbing stairs

Without use of rail or stick = 3, with use of
rail or stick = 2, unable to do = 1, unable to
assess = 0 ....

Up

Number of stairs ....
Time taken (sec) ....
Rating ....

Rolling

Without use of any aid = 3, with use of aid
= 2, unable to do = 1, unable to assess = 0

Right

Time taken (sec) ....
Rating ....

Left

Time taken (sec) ....
Rating ....

Lying to sitting

Scores 3-0 as for rolling
Time taken (sec) ....
Rating ....

Sitting to standing

Scores 3-0 as for rolling
Time taken (sec) ....
Rating ....

Dexterity

Able = 3, with assistance = 2, unable to do
= 1, unable to assess = 0
Fasten three shirt buttons — maximum time 3
minutes
Time taken (sec) ....
Rating ....

Getting up from floor

Without use of any aid = 3, with use of aid
= 2, unable to do = 1, unable to assess = 0
Time taken (sec) ....
Rating ....

Total score ....

The Yahr rating

This is a recognised scale to record overall
disease severity. It is as follows:

I   Uni-lateral involvement only, usually with
minimal or no functional impairment.
II Bi-lateral or midline involvement without
impairment of balance.
III First signs of impaired righting reflexes.
Functionally restricted in his activities but
can lead independent life. Disability mild
to moderate.
IV Severely disabled. Able to walk and stand
unaided, but is markedly handicapped.
V Confinement to bed or wheelchair unless
aided.

Handwriting sample

Write out name in full, *not* signature
Assessment 1 ....
Assessment 2 ....
Assessment 3 ....
Assessment 4 ....

Current anti-parkinsonian medication

Assessment 1 ....
Assessment 2 ....
Assessment 3 ....
Assessment 4 ....

Section Three
Treatment plan

Patient's problem	Therapist's aim	Plan of action	Starting date	Finishing date	Therapist's comments	Outcome rating Physiotherapist	Patient	Total no of sessions
1.								
2.								
3.								
4.								
5.								

* Outcome rating: Worse = 1, no change = 2, moderate improvement = 3, marked improvement = 4

Source: Franklyn 1986

with the Parkinson's Disease Society of Great Britain. The form of assessment is divided into three sections:

1. General information and medical history;
2. Physiotherapy assessment;
3. Treatment plan and outcome-rating.

Section one

The medical history includes the common symptoms of Parkinson's disease. It is advisable to ask the patient to name his symptoms rather than reading the list out to him. *Bradykinesia* is slowness of movement. *Pain* is fairly common, affecting the lumbar spine and thighs. When the patient is unable to move his feet, this is called *freezing*. Patients who have taken levodopa or similar drugs for some years may experience end-of-dose symptoms or the *on–off syndrome*, i.e. periods of very limited mobility or total immobility which may last from a few minutes to an hour or more. In these cases, it may prove helpful to complete section two on two separate occasions before treatment begins and use the mean of each pair of results as a base line.

Section two

To complete this part of the form, a stopwatch and a tape measure are required. In order to minimise the effects of drug-induced changes in performance on the assessment results, the assessments should take place at the same time of day and the time that has elapsed since the last dose of drugs should be noted. As it is important that past results do not influence the present assessment, the earlier records should be covered up during the assessment.

Posture. This can be affected in the early stages of the disease and so care should be taken to examine this while the patient is standing. The findings should be compared with the diagram shown on Fig. 4.1, p. 36. Allow the patient time to adopt his normal posture.

Balance. This is frequently affected as the disease progresses and may affect the amount and type of activity that a patient can perform. Scoring for this session is: YES = 2; NO = 1.

Activities. Most of the remaining assessment is concerned with activities that are commonly affected in Parkinson's disease. Any other that the assessor wishes to record should be named, timed and scored. Each activity is scored as follows:

3 = Able to complete the task without the use of an aid;
2 = Able to complete the task with the use of an aid;
1 = Unable to complete the task;
0 = Unable to assess.

At the end of an assessment, the scores of activities in section two can be totalled and compared with previous scores to give a quick assessment of the patient's performance. The maximum score is 24. For those activities that are timed, a stopwatch should be used. The timing should start when the patient has fully understood the task and is ready to start and should finish when the task has been fully completed.

Gait. Difficulty in initiating movement is a common problem. The normal heel–toes gait is often disturbed and the patient may walk with either a flat foot or a toe–heel gait. It is important to note this carefully. The number of strides and the time taken to complete the distance should be recorded. A fixed distance is not suggested for the latter measurement, but the distance chosen should be constant at each assessment. Loss of involuntary arm-swing when walking is on the affected side and should be noted (see Fig. 4.1, p. 37, point 5).

The Yahr rating. This rating as used here is an amended scale; a high-rating score in this assessment paper indicates disability.

Drug regimes. The drugs that are administered are often altered and this may affect performance, so it is important to note any change in medication.

Section three

This section contains the treatment plan and outcome ratings.

Flewitt-Handford exercises for parkinsonian gait. Handford (1986) describes a simple programme for activity that may be carried out in the patient's home. The aim of the exercises are to:

1. Re-teach heel strike — if patients are unable to get 90° active dorsiflexion at the ankle, a small heel-raise may be necessary;
2. Improve weight transference;

3. Increase the range of active movement at the knee and particularly the hip joints;
4. Move all the joints and muscles in the lower limb through the full range of movement to prevent secondary stiffness and weakness.

The exercises.

1. Long-sitting — alternate flexion/extension of the toes, feet and knees;
2. Crook-lying — rolling the knees from side to side;
3. Lying — alternate hip and knee flexion/extension, lifting each foot off the plinth;
4. Standing — facing and holding onto a chair to do the following:

   (a) to practise high-stepping;
   (b) with straight knees and not leaning backwards, to practise alternate feet dorsiflexion;
   (c) to cross the left leg in front of the right and vice versa, each time trying to touch the floor heel first;
   (d) to practise weight transference by walking sideways up and down parallel bars arranged at right angles to chair, to practise taking strides from toe off first the right leg and then the left leg or vice versa.

When walking, patients must learn to put their heels down first with every step. If a patient becomes 'stuck' while walking, he can become 'unstuck' by rocking backwards, so that weight is going through his heels. The patient then takes a step backwards and he will be able to move forwards again.

GEGENHALTEN OR PARATONIC RIGIDITY

This is a disorder seen in older patients and it is characterised by a resistance to passive movement by a counterpull which is present throughout the range of movement. It is often associated with dementia and apraxia and primitive reflexes such as pouting, grasping and sucking.

TARDIVE DYSKINESIA

Tardive dyskinesias are abnormal involuntary movements occurring most often in the oral region. The movements consist of puckering, chewing, sucking and darting movements of the tongue. Although they may be seen in patients who have not been on anti-psychotic agents, they are most commonly seen in patients treated with these agents. Metoclopramide can also cause these movements. They are more likely to occur in patients with previous brain damage and they can be extremely distressing for the patient. Choreoathetoid movements are seen less commonly.

PRIMITIVE REFLEXES

These reflexes are found normally in early infancy but disappear as the child matures. Their presence in old age indicates diffuse brain damage.

Grasp reflex

Stroking the palm of the hand produces flexion of the fingers with abduction of the thumb. The reflex is bilateral when brain damage is diffuse, but localised frontal-lobe damage after cerebrovascular accident may produce a unilateral reflex.

Sucking and pouting reflexes

Stroking the lips may produce a sucking movement and tapping the skin above the upper lip may cause pouting. Pouting and sucking reflexes may be observed in patients with diffuse brain damage and patients who have been on phenothiazine therapy for some time.

CERVICAL SPONDYLOSIS

Spondylosis is the commonest disorder of the cervical spine (Apley 1982) and in the elderly, radiographic evidence is almost universal, though many patients exhibit no neurological abnormality. The lower cervical discs degenerate and disc material extrudes;

surrounding fibrosis may spread to the root sleeves. The edges of the vertebral bodies hypertrophy (lipping) and later the intervertebral joints degenerate. The patient complains of neck pain which comes on gradually and is often worse on first getting up. The pain may radiate widely — to the occiput and frontal region, to the scapular muscles and down one or both arms. Paraesthesiae, weakness and clumsiness are occasionally symptoms. Osteophytes may distort the vertebral arteries and interfere with the blood supply to the hindbrain. As a result, transient ischaemic attacks may be brought on by neck movements, particularly extension and rotation.

The primary aim of physiotherapy will be to relieve the symptoms and to give the patient advice. The limiting factors which arise as a result of the pathology of the disease must be borne in mind when determining a suitable course of treatment. Lateral flexion will be severely limited due to fusion at the joints of Luschka; rotation and extension are movements that will tend to exacerbate symptoms and flexion is a deformity the physiotherapist attempts to avoid. The dilemma is that despite these factors, it is important to maintain as great a degree of mobility as possible. If pain is very severe, two to three days bed rest may be necessary. If the condition of the patient is suitable, traction may be tried when there is referred pain. However, it is essential to ensure that contraindications are not present, particularly osteoporosis. It is important that the patient is positioned so that he is comfortable and that the traction is arranged so that the traction force pulls the patient into a position that normally gives relief from pain; this will usually be one of flexion. Progression of traction is stopped once relief of symptoms is achieved. It should be remembered that relief of symptoms *during* treatment is not as relevant as the degree of relief maintained between treatment sessions.

The majority of patients with acute pain can be treated with a plastazote collar. The collar must fit correctly, be individually made and not be a 'neck warmer'. It must limit movement and hold the cervical spine in the correct posture. Patients quickly learn to rely on a collar which becomes an essential prop; encouragement must be towards wearing the collar less and less. Many patients are unaware of the effect that wearing a collar can have upon balance, especially at night when compensation offered by sight during daylight hours may not adequately compensate for the loss of joint and muscle receptor afferent information from the cervical spine. Patients should be advised to go out at night only if accompanied and warned of the possible effects that wearing a collar might have upon their balance.

Pain may be relieved by the application of heat in the form of infra-red or hot packs. Interferential therapy using a quadrupolar field and frequency of 90–100 Hz or 100–32 Hz is an effective and comfortable treatment.

Isometric muscle work may be given to the extensor muscles of the cervical spine, especially the short extensors. The patient is advised about sleeping posture and about daily activities such as shopping. The emphasis is placed on relaxation of the muscles around the shoulder girdle and on not putting excessive stress on the arms, for example by carrying shopping bags or dragging shopping trolleys.

Cervical myelopathy

Cervical spondylosis is the commonest cause of cervical cord compression in old age. In a postmortem study Brownell and Hughes (1975) found that 10 per cent of hospital subjects over the age of 70 had observable degeneration of the cervical cord due to spondylitic changes. Weakness and muscle wasting in the upper limbs are common symptoms and the patient may notice increasing clumsiness in performing tasks. Involvement of the lower limbs will lead to increasing difficulty in walking and examination reveals spastic paraparesis. Some patients do very well after surgical decompression, particularly if the condition is diagnosed before the patient becomes very immobile.

SUB-ACUTE COMBINED DEGENERATION OF THE CORD

Deficiency of Vitamin B_{12} may cause pathological changes in the spinal cord (dorsal columns) and peripheral nerves. Paraesthesiae of the feet and hands is an early feature and sensory loss may develop in the upper and lower limbs. The gait becomes progressively disordered with weakness, ataxia and spasticity. Pattie and Gilleard (1978) have emphasised that in the early stages of treatment, physiotherapy is crucial. They also stress that it is more important to adopt a multidisciplinary approach to the disabled person rather than spend time wrangling over the precise number of micrograms of Vitamin B_{12}.

MYASTHENIA GRAVIS

This disorder occasionally starts in the elderly, but usually not in the classic form of peripheral or ocular weakness that increases as the day progresses. The symptoms are mainly bulbar with loss of voice after talking for a few minutes and difficulty in getting through a meal because of impairment of chewing and swallowing. Ptosis is also common.

MOTOR NEURON DISEASE

Motor neuron disease usually affects men between 55 and 75 years of age. There is progressive muscle wasting. The upper limbs may be flaccid whilst the lower limbs may be spastic. Bulbar involvement leads to atrophy of the tongue, increasing dysphagia and dysarthria. Respiratory muscle involvement leads to breathing difficulties and often the terminal event is a chest infection. Nothing can be done at present to halt the progress of the disease and treatment is supportive. Particular emphasis must be placed on emotional and psychological comfort as the patient remains mentally alert during the illness.

DISORDERS OF THE AUTONOMIC NERVOUS SYSTEM

Degenerative changes in the autonomic nervous system produce a range of clinical manifestations, the most significant in the elderly being postural hypotension and hypothermia. Postural hypotension is discussed in Chapter 7. Because of abnormal central and peripheral thermoregulatory responses, a lowering of core temperature is more likely to occur in the elderly in a cold environment. Physiological protective mechanisms may be further impaired by illness and disability. All these factors place the elderly at particular risk of developing hypothermia. The risk of hypothermia is yet another reason why there must not be complacency about proper investigation and treatment of immobility in the elderly.

URINARY INCONTINENCE

Urinary incontinence is a common manifestation of illness in the older patient. As in other conditions, unless it is approached in a positive manner, treatable causes will be missed and the patient will endure unnecessary suffering. There are many causes of urinary incontinence in the elderly and the patient requires a detailed assessment.

The bladder is supplied by the automatic nervous system and it has a sympathetic and parasympathetic nerve supply. Stimulation of the sympathetic nerves causes contraction of the internal sphincter. Stimulation of the parasympathetic nerve causes relaxation of the internal sphincter, contraction of the detrusor muscle and emptying of the bladder. Local centres in the sacral cord are controlled by higher coordinating centres in the brain. Damage to these higher regulatory centres by conditions such as stroke or dementia will lead to an unstable bladder. The patient loses control of bladder function and is unable to inhibit micturition once the desire to void has been appreciated. Urge incontinence is a common feature of the early stages of stroke. In most patients it is transient but in a small minority it becomes intractable. An infarct in the right frontal lobe may involve the cortical centre for micturition control and result in a left hemiparesis with intractable urinary incontinence. Incontinence forms one of the characteristic triad of symptoms of internal hydrocephalus, together with confusion and gait apraxia. Damage to the spinal cord or to the sacral micturition reflex by surgery or disease will also lead to incontinence. The autonomic neuropathy associated with diabetes leads to an atonic bladder with chronic retention and overflow incontinence (Brocklehurst 1984).

Chronic retention of urine may be caused by local factors in the genitourinary system such as prostatic enlargement, urethral stricture, compression on the urethra due to faecal impaction and the effect of anti-cholinergic drugs. These drugs include tricyclic antidepressants, phenothiazines, and anti-parkinsonian agents. Chronic retention, if unrelieved, will result in overflow incontinence.

Urethral sphincter weakness results in incontinence whenever the pressure within the bladder exceeds the squeeze pressure of the urethra. Urethral closure mechanisms become less efficient with age in women and oestrogen deficiency appears to be an important factor. Damage during childbirth due to overstretching of the pelvic muscles and fascia may also weaken the closure mechanism.

Prostatectomy is a common cause of outlet weakness in the male. Patients with weak outlet mechanisms may become incontinent when they stand and this may be misinterpreted by the physiotherapist as a protest against exercising. When the patient stands, the weight of the abdominal contents increases the internal pressure of the bladder. Straining, coughing and lifting will produce stress incontinence through similar mechanisms. Urinary-tract infection may be an important aetiological factor if incontinence is of recent origin. Treatment of the infection has little influence on chronic incontinence.

Other factors

Poor mobility and lack of manual dexterity are common causes of incontinence. Defective vision may also contribute to it in some patients. Diuretic therapy may precipitate incontinence in a patient who previously has had full control. This is particularly likely to happen in patients with problems of mobility. Oversedation will also increase the likelihood of incontinence, particularly at night.

Very depressed patients may become incontinent through lack of motivation. Occasionally patients may use incontinence as a form of manipulation or protest when they feel they have no other effective way of expressing their disapproval or unhappiness.

Treatment

Treatment will obviously depend on the source or cause of the problem in the first instance. This is why it is so important that all patients are investigated as early as possible. Specific treatment such as prostatectomy or a gynaecological operation may be indicated. Oestrogen may be of value in women with weak, urethral-closure mechanisms.

Treatment of faecal impaction may relieve pressure on the urethra, thus relieving urinary incontinence. Faecal impaction due to constipation is also a common cause of faecal incontinence. Improving the patient's mobility will lessen the tendency to constipation. Pelvic-floor exercises are also useful for faecal incontinence.

Temporal voiding schedules (habit training) are frequently used to manage urinary incontinence. The patient is taken to void urine at definite intervals and it is noted on a chart if the patient is wet or dry at the time. The intervals are gradually adjusted until the patient is found to be dry when attended. Bladder training or bladder drill aims to correct the habit of frequent voiding and to improve voluntary control over the micturition reflex by gradually increasing the intervals between voiding. Drugs with anti-cholinergic properties are used in the management of patients with unstable bladders.

Physiotherapy

If the patient has problems with mobility or manual dexterity, physiotherapy may improve the situation dramatically even if there is another aetiological factor as well. Re-education of the muscles of the pelvic floor is one of the simplest and most rewarding methods of regaining bladder control for those with troublesome but not severe urinary incontinence. A number of studies have confirmed the success of physiotherapy as a safe, quick noninvasive technique (Hendrikson 1981; Harrison 1983; Castledene, Duffin and Mitchel 1984).

Electrical stimulation of the perineal muscles followed by exercise has been advocated for many years as a treatment for stress incontinence. The results inevitably depend upon the motivation of both patient and physiotherapist. Various types of electrical impulse can be used; the aim is to produce a maximum muscle contraction with minimum sensory discomfort. The older Faradic current has been replaced by pulses of variable duration and speed and interferential current. Wilson *et al.* (1984) were sceptical of the results of interferential current and exercise. However, Dougall (1986) reported a significant reduction in frequency and a 30 per cent reduction in the incidence of incontinence in the group treated. Sixty-five per cent of the group had maintained the improvement twelve months after the completion of treatment. Shepherd (1986), using a combination of electrical stimulation and an intensive re-education of the pelvic-floor muscles, showed improvement in 39 out of 44 women, including patients aged over 70.

The levator ani muscles, under voluntary control, possess the ability to stop voiding in mid-stream. These muscles have quick-twitch muscle fibres capable of responding rapidly and fatiguing quickly. Re-education of this group of muscles may be achieved by exercises alone. The peri-urethral muscles maintain the resting urethral tone and like the postural muscles of the body, this group is of slow-twitch type. They are capable of sustaining contraction and do not fatigue easily.

The first priority is to attempt to explain carefully to the patient the reason for re-education of the pelvic floor muscles and to make the patient aware of her perineum so that she can produce a

47

voluntary contraction. If two fingers are placed just within the introitus, the physiotherapist will be able to assess the presence of a muscle contraction. There are a number of ways of establishing good muscle control, but the emphasis should be on creating an awareness of a constant pelvic floor contraction which is maintained even during a cough.

Electrical stimulation

Interferential therapy

The patient is supported in a half-lying position and four large vacuum electrodes are used, two placed symmetrically on the abdomen above the inguinal ligaments and two placed on the medial side of the thighs below the inferior border of the femoral triangle (See Fig. 4.2). An interferential current of 0–100 Hz is passed between the electrodes. The intensity of the stimulation is taken to the maximum limit of patient comfort and tolerance. The treatment is given for 15 minutes, three times a week for four weeks. The method was first devised by McQuire (1975).

Figure 4.2: To show the position of electrodes in interferential therapy for incontinence

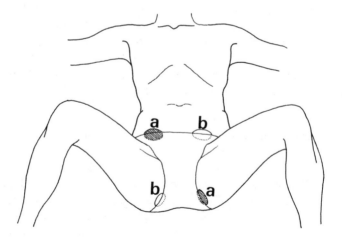

a. One set of paired electrodes
b. Alternate set of paired electrodes

Education (after Mandelstam 1986)

The patient is given a simple description of the pelvic floor and the aim of treatment is to re-educate the levator ani muscles. This is followed by digital examination to assess muscle tone. The patient is also instructed in the use of these muscles. Once initiated, the patient is encouraged to contract the muscles strongly four times. This is repeated frequently at convenient times. The patient is instructed:

1. To tighten and relax the muscles around the back passage;
2. While passing urine, to stop the flow and notice the sensation of muscle contraction in the front;
3. Once both these movements are learned, to start by contracting the back passage and then the front part. The pelvic muscles work as a whole and are to be contracted slowly four times. Repeat as often as possible.

After 2–3 weeks practice, there will be an awareness of the sensation of closure of the passages (back and front) and the feeling of drawing up the pelvic floor in front. The abdominal, thigh and buttock muscles should not be tightened and legs should remain uncrossed so that the pelvic muscles alone can be felt. It is a distinct and separate movement from the other muscles and can be checked by placing one finger into the vagina and contracting the muscles. It may be difficult to teach self-assessment to the over 65s because of lack of manual dexterity or because of cultural taboos. However, physiotherapists should be able to teach the technique should the opportunity arise. Exercises should be continued daily for three months.

Intractable incontinence

Some patients may not respond to either medical, surgical or physiotherapy treatment. A considerable amount can be done to keep these patients comfortable. There are many well-designed pads, pants, appliances and indwelling catheters available (Robinson 1982).

REFERENCES

Apley, A.G. (1982) 'The neck.' In A.G. Apley, (ed), *System of orthopaedics and fractures*, 6th Edn., Butterworth Scientific, London

Asher, R. (1947) 'The dangers of going to bed.' *Brit. Med. J. 253*, Dec. 13

Bowen, D.M. and Davison, A.N. (1982) 'The biochemistry of the ageing brain.' In F.I. Caird, (ed), *Neurological disorders in the elderly*, Wright, Bristol

Brocklehurst, J.C. (1984) *Urology in the elderly*, Churchill Livingstone, Edinburgh and New York

Brodie, B.B. and Shore, P.A. (1957) 'A concept for a role of serotonin and norepinephrine as chemical mediators in the brain.' *Ann. N.Y. Acad. Sci., 66*, 631

Brody, H. (1982) 'Age changes in the nervous system.' In F.I. Caird (ed) *Neurological disorders in the elderly*, Wright, Bristol

Brownell, B. and Hughes, H.T. (1975) 'Degeneration of muscle in association with carcinoma of the bronchus.' *J. Neurol. Neurosurg. Psychiatry, 38* (4), 363–70

Campbell, M.J. and McComas, A.J. (1977) 'Physiological changes in ageing muscles.' *J. Neurol. Neurosurg. Psychiatry, 36* (2), 174–82

Castledene, C.M., Duffin, H.M. and Mitchel, F.P. (1984) 'The effect of physiotherapy in stress incontinence.' *Age and Ageing 13*, 235–7

Coakley, D. and Snell, A. (1979) 'Unrecognised fractures in old age.' *Practitioner, 223*, (1338) 828–9

Cotzias, G.C., Van Woert, M.H. and Schiffer, L.M. (1967) 'Aromatic amino acids and modification in parkinsonism.' *New Eng. J. Med., 276*, 374

Dougall, D.S. (1985) 'The effects of interferential therapy on incontinence and frequency of micturition.' *Physiotherapy, 71*, 3, 135–6

Franklyn, S. (1986) 'User's guide to the physiotherapy assessment form for Parkinson's disease.' *Physiotherapy, 72*, 7, 359–61

Gutman, E. and Hanzlikova, V. (1966) 'Motor unit old age.' *Nature, 290*, 921–2

Handford, F. (1986) 'The Flewitt-Handford exercises for parkinsonian gait.' *Physiotherapy, 77*, 8, 382

Harrison, M.A. (1982) 'Parkinsonism.' In P.A. Downie (ed), *Cash's textbook of neurology for physiotherapists*, Faber and Faber, London

Harrison, S.M. (1983) 'Stress incontinence and the physiotherapist.' *Physiotherapy 69*, 3, 144–7

Hendrikson, L.S. (1981) 'The frequency of stress incontinence in women before and after the implementation of an exercise program.' *Issues in Health Care of Women, 3*, 81–92

Hildick-Smith, M. (1979) 'Parkinsonism — careful assessment the key.' *Geriat. Med., 9*, 4, 70

—————— (1979) 'Parkinsonism – a time to evaluate therapy.' *Geriat. med., 9*, 5, 22

Kinnear, E. (1986) 'Long-term management of Parkinson's disease.' *Physiotherapy, 72*, 7, 340–1

McQuire, W.A. (1975) 'Electrotherapy and exercises for stress incontinence and frequency.' *Physiotherapy, 61*, 10, 305–7

Mandelstam, D. (1986) *Incontinence and Its Management*, 2nd edn, Croom Helm, London and New York

Pattie, A.H. and Gilleard, C.J. (1978) 'Admission and adjustment of residents in homes for the elderly.' *J. Epidemiol. Community Health, 32* (3), 212–4

Robinson, J.M. (1982) 'The management of urinary incontinence.' In D. Coakley and V.J. Hanson (eds), *Nursing and the Doctor*, Pitman, London

Rowe, R.W.D. (1969) 'The effect of sensibility on skeletal muscles in the mouse.' *Exp. Gerontol., 4*, 119–26

Shepherd, A.M. (1986) 'Re-education of the muscles of the pelvic floor.' In D. Mandelstam (ed), *Incontinence and its management*, 2nd edn, Croom Helm, London

Wale, J.O. (1961) 'Diseases of the sensory neurons.' In J.O. Wale (ed), *Tidy's massage and remedial exercises*, Wright, Bristol

Wilson, P.D., Al Samarrac, T., Deakin, M., Kolbe, E. and Brown, A.D.G. (1984) 'The value of physiotherapy in female genuine stress incontinence.' *Proc. Int. Continence Soc.* (Innsbruck), 156–8

5

The Management of Stroke

SECTION ONE

A stroke may be defined as an acute disturbance of cerebral function of vascular origin causing disability lasting more than, or death within, 24 hours. If the disability does not last more than 24 hours, the episode is described as a transient ischaemic attack. Seventy-five per cent of all strokes occur in patients over the age of 65, with an annual incidence of 18 per 1,000 population compared with an annual incidence of 2 per 1,000 population at all ages. Stroke is, therefore, very much an illness of old age. One in every eight hospital beds (excluding maternity beds and beds in psychiatric hospitals) in Scotland is occupied by a stroke patient. If current trends continue, it has been projected that no less than 18 per cent of all available hospital beds will be taken up by stroke patients by the end of this century (Akhtar and Garroway 1982). Stroke is the leading cause of disability in the Western world and there are approximately a million new cases in Europe every year.

Risk factors

Most of the information about risk factors relates to patients under the age of 60. Factors that have been implicated in younger adults include race, social class, high blood pressure, obesity, elevated serum cholesterol, cigarette smoking, vascular disease, raised haematocrit and diabetes.

One cannot necessarily extrapolate the findings of stroke studies in younger adults to the elderly. For instance, a high level of serum cholesterol has been related to stroke in early adult life but there does not appear to be a relationship between stroke and cholesterol levels in older patients. In an American study, cigarette smoking was found to be a significant aetiological factor for strokes in older patients, but this finding was not confirmed in an English study. Diabetes and impaired glucose tolerance are associated with increased risk of stroke in younger patients, but as yet it is uncertain whether adequate control of glucose intolerance decreases the incidence of stroke in old age (Evans and Caird 1982).

Hypertension is one of the most significant risk factors for stroke in the elderly. The decision whether to treat high blood pressure or not in this age group has always been a controversial issue. A recent major European study of stroke in the elderly found a reduction in stroke, congestive cardiac failure and fatal myocardial infarction in patients treated with anti-hypertensive therapy (Amery *et al.* 1985).

Untreated transient ischaemic attacks lead to cerebral infarction in 15 to 25 per cent of cases. However, there is also a very high risk of serious heart disease in these patients and they are more likely to die from cardiac problems than from stroke. The majority of transient ischaemic attacks are thought to be due to embolisation of platelet, fibrin or atheromatous debris from atherosclerotic plaques in the neck vessels. The neurological deficit is transient because the emboli are fragmented rapidly. Some patients with transient ischaemic attacks have marked stenosis in either the carotid or vertebrobasilar arteries. There are a number of conditions such as cardiac arrythmias, endocarditis, degenerative changes in the mitral valve and arteritis which can cause transient attacks. All patients should be investigated carefully. Whether patients with transient ischaemic attacks due to carotid problems should be treated medically with agents such as anti-coagulants and anti-platelet drugs or surgically is still very controversial. There are a number of controlled trials taking place at the moment and hopefully the results of these trials will give clearer guidance on the most appropriate treatment of these patients.

Site of the lesion

The majority of strokes are caused by lesions in the left or right cerebral hemispheres and about 20 per cent are due to brain-stem lesions. A lesion in the cerebral hemisphere will manifest itself clinically by neurological signs on the opposite side of the body. The brain is a very complex organ and the signs will depend on the region of the brain disrupted by the stroke. Damage to the motor area just in front of the fissure of Rolando will produce paralysis. Sensory changes will be produced by damage to the sensory area posterior to the same fissure. Most people (including the majority of left-handed people) have their speech centres on the left side of the brain. Damage to the speech centre (Broca's area) will lead to expressive dysphasia and the patient will experience difficulty in initiating speech. Damage to the speech area in the temporal lobe (as opposed to the frontal lobe) leads to a receptive dysphasia and the patient cannot make sense of what is being said to him. Clinically it is uncommon to see a patient with pure receptive or expressive dysphasia. There is usually a combination of expressive and receptive features, although one pattern may be dominant. Apart from dysphasia, damage to the frontal lobe can produce agraphia (difficulty in writing). As might be expected, damage to the temporal lobe, which is concerned more with 'reception', may cause difficulty in reading or dyslexia. Lesions of the frontal area also cause changes in personality and disorders in mood. The patient usually has emotional lability and will laugh or cry quite inappropriately. This can be very distressing for relatives particularly if the condition has not been explained to them.

Parietal lobe damage on the left side of the brain leads to an inability to calculate (acalculia). Constructional ability may be impaired and this may be tested by asking the patient to draw something such as a house. The patient may also experience difficulty in dressing. Damage to the right parietal lobe leads to problems with perception. The patient may ignore his hemiplegic side and if the lesion extends towards the occipital area, he may also ignore the left visual field (visual inattention). Destruction in this area of the brain can be very disabling as the perceptual problems are a major barrier in rehabilitation. Visual-field loss occurs when the optic radiation or occipital lobe is damaged. The usual presentation being loss of vision towards the hemiplegic side (homonymous hemianopia).

Motor neurons leave the hemispheres through the pathways known as the internal capsules. Sensory fibres ascend through the same narrow gateway. Small lesions here can cause disabling strokes. Similarly, lesions in the brain stem can also disrupt the motor and sensory neurons, leading to a stroke. As the reticular formation, which regulates consciousness, is also in the brain stem, the patient may be deeply unconscious. If the cerebellum and the brain stem are involved, the patient will have problems with his co-ordination and may be ataxic.

From this brief summary it is clear that a stroke can present in many ways and all patients must be carefully assessed to determine the full extent of their disabilities.

Pathophysiology

Although there is considerable variation in the mode of presentation, the basic pathophysiology of stroke can be divided into two main groups — those caused by cerebral infarction and those caused by cerebral haemorrhage.

Cerebral infarction

Over 80 per cent of strokes are due to cerebral infarction. The oxygen supply of the neurons is suddenly interrupted leading to cell death. This may be caused by thrombosis in the carotid or vertebral arteries or in their branches in the brain. However, it is now recognised that emboli from a source in the large vessels supplying the brain or in the heart itself are an important cause of cerebral infarction, particularly in the elderly. Small areas of infarction (known as lacunes) can be produced by thrombosis within micro-aneurysms, which are often present in the brains of elderly hypertensive patients. If these small lesions are strategically placed, they can produce focal neurological signs such as a pure motor stroke or a pure sensory stroke. Lacunes are found mostly in the basal ganglia, internal capsule, thalamus and brain stem.

It is now recognised that hypotensive episodes may also lead to cerebral infarction in elderly patients. The control of cerebral blood flow is impaired in the elderly and a sudden drop in blood pressure may cause infarction in an area of the brain where the blood supply is already compromised.

Cerebral haemorrhage

Cerebral haemorrhage accounts for about 20 per cent of stroke cases. In older people, the majority of strokes are due to rupture of a microaneurysm within the cerebral tissue. However, subarachnoid haemorrhages also occur in older patients and about 8 per cent of strokes are caused by them.

Investigations

Apart from the usual routine investigations such as haemoglobin, erythrocyte sedimentation rate, blood glucose, etc., which may reveal valuable information, there are a number of more specialised procedures that may be carried out.

Brain scan

This technique has the advantage of being non-invasive. The brain is scanned after the intravenous injection of a synthetic radio-isotope. It is particularly useful if a brain tumour or subdural haematoma is suspected. Cerebral infarcts cannot be seen in the early stages in the brain scan.

Computerised axial tomography

This is another non-invasive technique and its development marked a great advance in the investigation of stroke disease. It not only identifies the site of the lesion accurately, but also identifies its nature. Cerebral infarction is shown as a low-density area and it becomes detectable within the first day of the stroke. Cerebral haemorrhage shows as a high-density area. CAT scanning will also identify other lesions such as brain tumours and subdural haematomas.

Angiography

An arteriogram demonstrates the blood vessels of the brain and identifies problem areas within them. It is an invasive technique involving an injection of contrast media into the intra-arterial system and it is not without danger. It is only indicated when there is a definite possibility of surgery.

Ultrasound

Ultrasound (phonoangiography) is used as a non-invasive method when investigating disease in the neck vessels of patients with stroke or threatened stroke. Modern equipment can give very good results even when compared with more invasive methods. Ultrasound is particularly valuable as a screening technique.

Home or hospital

Admission to hospital makes it easier to investigate the acute stroke so that remediable conditions are diagnosed promptly. However, in some areas only 40 per cent of patients are admitted to hospital on the first day of stroke (Brocklehurst *et al.* 1978) and the decision whether to admit or not appears to be governed by social factors. Patients with minor strokes and transient attacks could be investigated on a day-care basis provided that this can be done promptly. The day hospital can play a useful role in this situation. Some families may wish to keep aged relatives with a stroke and poor prognosis at home and this should be facilitated. Some would argue that all other stroke patients should be admitted initially to hospital, whilst others argue that many of these patients can be managed adequately at home. If home care is to be effective, facilities must be good with adequate medical and nursing cover, domiciliary physiotherapy and occupational therapy.

Management

Many stroke patients are either unconscious or very drowsy when first admitted. Careful attention must be given to maintaining a patent airway in these patients and in those with bulbar palsy. A nasogastric tube should be inserted and intravenous fluids may be necessary in the first 48 hours. Urine output must be monitored carefully. Condom or catheter drainage may be necessary in some patients.

The physiotherapist should be involved at this early stage and should advise the team about the most appropriate methods of positioning the patient. Figures 5.1–5.4 (pp. 58–61) show the positions used in nursing patients following a cerebrovascular accident. In the early stages, passive movements of the paralysed limbs can be carried out when the patient's position is being changed. Chest physiotherapy may also be necessary to treat or prevent respiratory infections.

The prevention of pressure sores is an important aspect of supportive care and this subject is discussed in Chapter 9.

Reassurance and explanation

A stroke is a catastrophic experience for a patient and his relatives. They will need considerable reassurances and the physiotherapist should offer support whenever possible. She is going to have a one-

Figure 5.1: Lying supine

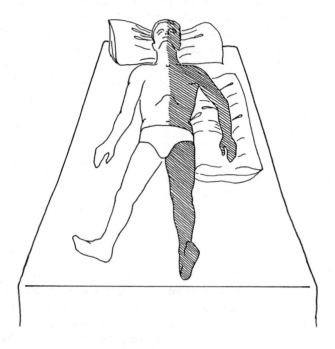

Head and neck in neutral position or turned to the affected side
Affected arm protracted at the shoulder
Elbow extended and supported on a pillow
Fingers in as extended a position as it is possible to achieve
Trunk elongated on the affected side
Pillow placed under the pelvis to prevent rotation of the hip on the
affected side
NOTHING in contact with the palm of the hand or the sole of the foot.

to-one working relationship with the patient and, if she can convey
to the patient that she has an understanding of the terrible crisis he
is experiencing, then she is more likely to receive co-operation
during therapy. At the earliest opportunity, the patient should be
given a careful explanation of what has happened to him and the
treatment programme should be outlined. This explanation should be
repeated on a number of occasions and more detail can be given as
the patient improves.

Figure 5.2: Side-lying on the affected side

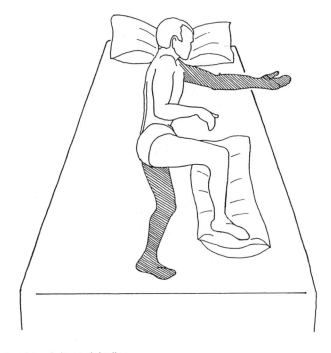

Head and trunk in straight line
Affected shoulder protracted; elbow extended; radio-ulnar joints
supinated
Affected leg extended at the hip and slight flexion at the knee
The unaffected (upper) leg placed in front of the other and supported on
a pillow
NOTHING in contact with the palm of the hand or the sole of the foot

Specific medical therapy

There are many uncertainties about the use of specific agents to treat
stroke in the acute phase. Trials of different agents in the past were
often inadequate and the results conflicting. One of the major
reasons for difficulty was the failure to differentiate between the
different causes of stroke when conducting trials. For instance, it is
quite likely that a good treatment for cerebral infarction would not
be effective in cerebral haemorrhage. Modern advances in investigation techniques now make it possible to look more critically at many
agents advocated in the past as treatments for stroke.

Figure 5.3: Side-lying on unaffected side

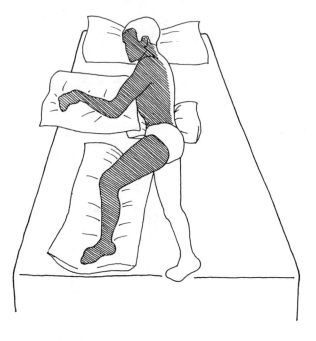

Patient in full side-lying
Head and trunk in straight line, with pillow under waist to elongate trunk
Shoulder protracted; elbow extended and supported on a pillow
Affected leg protracted at pelvis; slight flexion at the hip and knee
Foot must NOT overhang the pillow (i.e. supported on the pillow)

It was thought that drugs which would dilate the blood vessels of the brain (vasodilators) would be of value by increasing the blood flow to the ischaemic area. However, in practice, the reverse occurred, the damaged vessels did not dilate but the vessels in the rest of the brain did and blood was diverted from the ischaemic to the normal areas.

Cerebral oedema

If deterioration occurs immediately after a stroke, it is most likely to be due to progression of the stroke itself. However, if the patient deteriorates between the second and seventh days, it is most likely

Figure 5.4: Seated

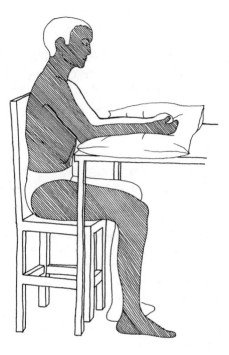

The patient must sit well back into the chair with hips, knees and ankles at 90°
Feet well supported on the floor
Weight evenly distributed on both buttocks
Both arms protracted forwards and supported on a table placed in front of the patient

due to cerebral oedema. The damaged brain swells and presses on the brain stem causing a gradual deepening of coma. A number of agents are used in attempts to control this cerebral oedema such as steroids, mannitol and glycerol. Again as in other areas of stroke treatment, there is no general agreement on the efficacy of the agents and we will have to await further research for clarification.

Complications

Death after the first week is likely to be due to complications such as bronchopneumonia or pulmonary embolus secondary to deep-vein thrombosis.

Bronchopneumonia

Bronchopneumonia may be prevented by chest physiotherapy and by encouraging the patient to cough. Good positioning of the patient and early mobilisation also help to prevent chest infections. In the unconscious patient, regular suction will be necessary to remove secretions.

Deep-vein thrombosis

This complication is most likely to occur about ten days after a stroke. The physiotherapist may be the first to notice the clinical signs — tenderness and swelling of the calf on the affected side which may feel warmer than the opposite calf. Venous thrombosis can occur, however, in the absence of clinical signs. About 50 per cent of patients develop a deep-vein thrombosis and it usually occurs in the paralysed limb. They can occur despite physiotherapy (including leg and breathing exercises) and in spite of a policy of early mobilisation. Prolonged pressure on the calf leading to damage to the vein wall is likely to be a significant factor in initiating thrombosis (Warlow 1978). Pulmonary embolus is the life-threatening complication of deep-vein thrombosis. The wearing of elastic stockings has been used as a preventive measure and in recent years, research has indicated that the incidence of deep-vein thrombosis can be reduced by the use of prophylactic, low-dose subcutaneous heparin. The low-dose regime provides protection without interfering with the clotting mechanism of the body (McCarthy *et al*. 1977).

SECTION TWO

In the previous section, the aetiology of stroke and its management during the acute phase were discussed. It was seen that the physiotherapist has a definite role in this early period. The physiotherapist becomes more involved as the emphasis on rehabilitation increases. However, the problems of the stroke patient are usually very complex and multiple so other professional workers, such as speech therapists and occupational therapists, will also be involved in working with the patient. A detailed assessment should be made by members of the multidisciplinary team so that the patient's potential can be assessed and any barriers to rehabilitation will be recognised.

This latter aspect is extremely important as, unless these barriers are identified, appropriate action to overcome them cannot be taken. Adams (1974) identified six criteria for basic assessment:

1. Exercise tolerance;
2. Motivation;
3. Sensory impairment;
4. Mental capacity;
5. Motor deficit;
6. Postural control.

Exercise tolerance

Poor exercise tolerance can be a big problem in elderly patients as many suffer from conditions other than stroke, such as cardiac or respiratory disease and arthritis. Tolerance may also be impaired by postural hypotension and all older patients who are being mobilised should have their blood pressure checked on lying and standing. Should the therapist remain unaware of the problem, the patient may be unable to co-operate and may fall.

Motivation

Poorly motivated patients may improve if reassured and encouraged. Some patients may be depressed and it is often worth a trial of anti-depressant therapy when this is suspected.

Sensory or perceptual problems

Patients with damage to the parietal lobe can have very marked perceptual problems. Difficulties with perception and proprioception can be major barriers in the way of progress. Some patients have gross disturbances of body image and they may neglect and even disown the affected part of the body. Little progress will be made unless the patient can be made aware of the problem. Similarly hemianopia and visual inattention may impede rehabilitation. Some patients not only have hemianopia but also ignore completely anything in the affected field of vision. These patients usually have a left hemiplegia and when asked to draw a house or clock for instance, they will draw only the right side. They may also only eat the food on the right side of their plates; this phenomenon is known as anosognosia.

A detailed assessment of sensation in the limbs should be carried out, testing for tactile sensation and proprioception. Problems of the parietal lobe may become apparent if there is inattention on one side when both sides are stimulated simultaneously. Other tests for cortical impairment include two-point discrimination and the ability to recognise the shape, size and texture of objects when the eyes are closed. Failure to do the latter is known as astereognosis.

Deafness

Deafness may also impede progress, particularly if the physiotherapist has not identified the problem in the early stages. It may be that a patient had a hearing aid before the stroke and that it was not brought into hospital. The hearing impairment may be simply due to wax in the ear and if the doctors are not aware of the patient's problem, it should be drawn to their attention so that the situation can be assessed. The difficulty may be one of comprehension rather than hearing and the patient may respond to mime when he cannot follow oral or written instructions.

Memory impairment

Patients may not only have problems in receiving and interpreting information after stroke, but they may also have problems in retaining it. Repetition is necessary, especially in the early stages. Memory may improve gradually but it is often one of the last aspects of intellectual impairment to return to normal after a stroke. Memory loss may, of course, be due to a pre-existing dementia (history from relatives) and this would be a major barrier to rehabilitation.

Apraxia

Apart from the obvious loss of voluntary motor power and the gradual development of spasticity after stroke, the patient may develop good power but be unable to accomplish a purposeful movement because of apraxia. Apraxia is present when the patient cannot carry out a previously established pattern of movement even though muscle power, sensation and co-ordination appear to be unimpaired. The difficulty is not a problem of comprehension because the patient will make appropriate verbal responses about the movement. He may, for instance, be unable to walk even though he can move both lower limbs independently.

Postural control

Failure to regain postural control is a bad prognostic sign for ultimate recovery. The patient who, some weeks after a stroke, cannot sit upright in the bed or chair without sliding to one side even when propped with cushions, usually makes very slow progress.

Physiotherapy management

It is essential that the physiotherapist should start treatment as soon as the vital signs are stable. Too often, a patient's functional outlook is ruined because of neglect in the early stages. In the rehabilitation of a stroke victim, 'to wait and see' is often disastrous. Carr and Shepherd (1979) place emphasis on four essential points:

1. The way in which motor skills are learned: repetition; practice; concentration;
2. The manner in which everyday movements are performed;
3. The importance of sensory feedback;
4. The relationship between motivation and learning.

A physiotherapist must appreciate the devastating shock to a patient when without prior warning, he is denied the functional use of one half of the body and may not be able to communicate. The fear alone of such a situation, quite apart from the pathology, may make the patient depressed, irritable and aggressive. All initial contacts with the patient must be positive and effective so that he may come to terms with an overwhelmingly stressful situation.

In order to appreciate how re-education or relearning might be approached, it is helpful to consider how education and learning are first realised in a child. Initially activities are learned in a sequence. They have to be relearned in a similar sequence, but with the added benefit of some previous experience. For example, the movement from the seated to the standing position involves a sequence of events: the feet are brought back, the head is pushed forwards and the trunk moves forwards from the hips. Not until the weight of the body is over the feet can the legs and trunk be extended. It is only possible to achieve this movement if accurate sensory feedback is present. Movements that a patient is relearning need to be broken down into basic patterns and part-patterns and each part practised repeatedly.

At the present time, there is a diversity of opinion as to the method of care of stroke patients. The prognosis of a patient may be such that little success may be achieved despite the best early rehabilitation. The number of patients that do progress to a modified functional independence may be small in relation to the total number of stroke victims. However, such patients must be given the opportunity to reach their maximal potential. They may develop their own adaptations to movement, which they feel are adequate, but which could result in maintaining spastic patterns and put unnecessary strain on already laboured movements.

The characteristic feature of hemiplegia is the loss of voluntary movement with alteration in muscle tone and sensation throughout one side of the body. Not only is there loss of power, but also of normal movement patterns, resulting in the presence of associated reactions (Cash 1974). Initially, a stage of hypotonus may exist which does not allow movement to be initiated. This normally gives way to hypertonus. If spasticity is severe, no movement at all will be possible. Moderate spasticity will allow only slow and abnormally co-ordinated movements to be performed with great effort. Normal co-ordination with respect to gross movements will be formed in cases of mild spasticity, but fine selective movements of individual limb segments will be impossible or performed slowly and clumsily.

Movement needs a constantly changing background of postural changes. Posture should be seen as temporarily arrested movement rather than as a static position, requiring interplay of muscle tone and regulated sensory feedback. The stereotyped static patterns of spasticity dominate and limit a patient's motor activity. Bobath (1970) has shown the effects of spasticity and how it interferes with every normal movement. One of the concerns of the physiotherapist therefore should be to control or lessen spasticity in order that the patient might regain more normal movements and use of the affected part.

In rehabilitation of relearning it is necessary to:

1. *Identify a goal.* To obtain a patient's co-operation and allay his undoubted confusion, an explanation of his situation must be given to him. To be realistic, a goal must not seem too far away.

2. *Inhibit unnecessary activity.* Basmajian, Regenous and Baker (1977) have shown that both development of motor co-ordination in childhood and acquisition of skills in adult life depend more on progressive inhibition of undesired muscle activity and unwanted responses, than on activation of additional motor units.

3. *Restore balance.* Balance is the state in which one's body is in equilibrium with the centre of gravity over a base of support. Balance is dynamic and requires sensory feedback to inform the body of minor changes in position. Subconscious balance control allows the body to perform isolated fine-motor skills in separate areas of the body whilst maintaining overall posture.

4. *Maintain body alignment.* There is an inherent 'central programming' unit in the brain which monitors movement and posture by checking the feedback signals with expectation that results from previous experience.

5. *Practice.* Practice is the key to any learning and one practises movement from childhood through the developmental sequence to adult life. A recognisable goal is always the aim. Mental practice, that is, rehearsing in the mind what is trying to be learned, is thought to aid muscular activity, provided anxiety is removed or avoided. This is only suitable for patients who do not have communication or perceptual problems.

6. *Develop motivation.* It is essential for a patient to motivate himself to aspire to the goal set within his own limitations. Positive reinforcement for actions achieved is important, but should be given at appropriate times and not used too frequently, as then there is the likelihood that it will lose its effectiveness.

7. *Use knowledge of results and feedback.* Sensory feedback via the patient's external senses and internal proprioceptors is vital when achievements have been made. Carr *et al.* (1970) comment that feedback consists of three parts:

(a) Internal feedback — a feed-forward mechanism, which signals an intended action, occurring prior to the action;
(b) Feedback proper — from the effector system during action;
(c) Knowledge of results occurring after the action is completed.

From this it may be seen that sensory feedback is essential in rehabilitation of smooth, controlled movement. Perceptual influences exert a great influence on a patient's movement difficulties and must never be forgotten. It is extremely difficult to cope with the patient who denies that the affected side exists. Where sensory and motor problems co-exist, they must both be treated with equal importance.

Techniques of treatment

Many books have been written on the topic of how to treat a hemiplegic patient. The advantages of the main methods are summarised here.

Bobath method

In the past, the standard treatment for hemiplegics was to introduce a short-term programme of compensatory rehabilitation to the unaffected side. This neglected the potential of the affected side and increased spasticity and decreased activity of that side. The Bobath technique is based on the theory that lesion of an upper motor neuron results in the release of abnormal tonic reflexes; these reflexes, which are progressively inhibited in childhood to allow normal postural reactions to develop, now produce abnormal movement synergies. The greater the degree of spasticity, the more lasting will be the associated reactions.

The changing state of the body musculature is constantly reflected in the distribution of excitatory and inhibitory processes within the central nervous system. Therefore, by changing the relative positions of the body and limbs, one can change postural patterns and hope to stop overflow into abnormal mass synergies. The patient should not be allowed to use basic limb synergies of flexion and extension, nor must the effect of tonic neck reflexes and other attitudinal reflexes be worked to facilitate or inhibit movements. Attempts must be made from the beginning to develop normal motor responses.

The aim of the Bobath approach, fully detailed in her book, 'Adult Hemiplegia: Evaluation and Treatment' (second edn., 1978, Heinemann), is to reduce spasticity by counteracting its abnormal patterns. Bobath accordingly developed movement patterns which not only inhibit abnormal postural reactions but, at the same time, facilitate active automatic and voluntary movements. The use of such patterns indicates active dynamic movement whereby the therapist inhibits spasticity and facilitates movement by guiding specific parts of the pattern. Using 'key points' of control situated proximally at the neck, spine, shoulder and pelvis, tone can be controlled and reduced distally. Toes, ankles, fingers and wrists can often be used as distal points of control to reduce spasticity proximally. Assessment plays a vital role in determining how the individual patient is best treated. Assessment of joint range and muscle power are worthless if control is variable through constantly fluctuating degrees of spasticity. Progression is made only when the patient can achieve the movements required without associated reactions. Bobath, in keeping with the inhibition-facilitation approach, establishes what abnormal movements need to be inhibited and what normal movements can be relied on during treatment with each particular patient. The following points summarise the main features of the technique:

1. Assessment of a patient's abnormal movement patterns must continue during treatment, becoming part of treatment;
2. Spasticity is reduced by reflex inhibiting postures;
3. Mass synergies and associated reactions must be avoided;
4. Balance and righting reactions are facilitated;
5. Voluntary activity is only enlisted when the patient can control the movement without effort or producing spasticity;
6. Sensory-motor re-education is facilitated;
7. Patient awareness and feedback are essential — repetition is an essential part of learning;
8. The untapped potential of the affected side is developed to the fullest possible extent.

Brunnstrom approach

Brunnstrom developed a special interest in patients with neuro-muscular disorders in the years after the Second World War. Her treatment is based upon the principle that voluntary movement develops as a product of more primitive reflexes modified in a particular sequence (Hughes 1972).

Brunnstrom determined that basic synergies found in hemiplegic patients are positive spinal-cord patterns that are retained throughout the evolutionary process. In spastic hemiplegia, they retain their positive stereotyped character. When the influence of higher centres is interfered with, pathological reflexes appear: these should be considered 'normal' because they were present during an earlier evolutionary period. Brunnstrom, in contradiction to Bobath, believes that during the early recovery phase the hemiplegic patient should be aided and encouraged to gain control of basic limb synergies. Once these limb synergies can be performed, a modification of the synergies brings out movement combinations which deviate from the synergies. The therapist conditions, modifies and inhibits the synergistic patterns using associated reactions, tonic neck reflexes, tonic labyrinthine reflexes, inter-facilitation and manual resistance.

Brunnstrom (1970) in her book, 'Movement Therapy in Hemiplegia', notes the recovery sequence in six stages:

1. Flaccidity following the acute episode;
2. Basic limb synergies or some of their components may appear as associated reactions or minimal voluntary movement responses may be present — spasticity develops;
3. The patient may gain voluntary control in small range — spasticity develops further and may become severe;
4. Some movement combinations that do not follow the paths of either synergy are mastered, first with difficulty, then with more ease and spasticity begins to decline;
5. If progress continues, more difficult movement combinations are learned as the basic limb synergies lose their dominance over motor activity;
6. Spasticity disappears — individual joint movements become possible and co-ordination approaches normal.

Brunnstrom developed her approach specifically for the hemiplegic patient. It is an attempt to provide a wedge between subcortical and cortical control. Her treatment is based on the principle that voluntary movement is a product of more primitive reflexes modified in a particular sequence. She uses abnormal synergies and reflex mechanisms to elicit movement.

The approach for any situation is as follows:

1. If voluntary movement is not present in any position or movement combination, a contraction is elicited reflexly;
2. The patient superimposes his voluntary effort on the reflex contraction;
3. Local facilitatory measures are introduced to reinforce the patient's voluntary effort;

4. Attempts are made to cause the muscle groups that have not been activated to respond in the desired situation.

Proprioceptive neuromuscular facilitation techniques (PNF)

The techniques of proprioceptive neuromuscular facilitation (PNF) were developed at the Kabat-Kaiser Institute in California between 1946 and 1951. Kabat's ideas were expanded by Knott and Voss (1973). The philosophy of PNF is based on the concept that life is a series of responses to a series of demands. Techniques of PNF therefore consist of placing a demand where a response is desired. PNF recognises that hidden potentials may exist that can be developed by response to demand and that frequency or repetition of activity is important to the learning process and to the development of endurance. 'Stronger' parts of the body are utilised to stimulate and strengthen 'weaker' parts, leading to a goal of optimum function.

Mass movement is a characteristic of normal motor activity and is in keeping with Beever's axiom that the brain knows nothing of individual muscle action but knows only of movement. Mass-movement patterns are spiral and diagonal in character. Each pattern is a three-component motion with respect to all joints or pivots of action participating in the movement. The components include:

1. Flexion or extension;
2. Motion towards and across the mid-line or across and away from the mid-line (adduction and abduction);
3. Rotation (medial or lateral).

The spiral and diagonal patterns provide for optimal contraction of the muscles involved. As a pattern is initiated, rotation occurs first at the spiral characteristic and the other two components combine to give the pattern a diagonal direction.

In dealing with the hemiplegic, whose main problem is the presence of spasticity and abnormal patterns of movement, certain considerations are noted:

1. Manual contact may be helpful in creating an awareness of the affected side especially if sensory loss is great;
2. Verbal commands combined with vision may act as a compensatory mechanism where dyspraxia exists;
3. Approximation is used to stimulate postural reflexes and is used only on weight-bearing joints;

4. Normal timing allows for re-establishment of sequence and assists the stroke patient through the process of learning and timing that establishes co-ordinated movements;

5. Stretch involves the danger of initiating a tonic reflex and moving into a total synergic pattern;

6. Maximum resistance may cause overflow of muscle activity into the spastic pattern of tonic contraction;

7. Reinforcement may only be used with great care to avoid the chance of increasing tone;

8. Patterns of movement, the essential ingredient of PNF are generally not suitable because they are mass movements that move into the area of synergic patterns of contraction. Because one of the components is a movement across or away from the mid-line, it is sometimes wrongly assumed that these movements will assist in re-education of postural reflexes and loss of body image. PNF should only be used to facilitate those muscles or groups of muscles that are opposed to the spastic pattern (Johnstone 1976).

Voss (1967) stated that the following techniques may be used to hasten motor learning:

1. Rapid repetitive stretching for initiation of voluntary movement and improving rhythm;

2. Resistance-graded so as to encourage range;

3. Approximation for activation of postural responses;

4. Combining movements for reinforcement;

5. Reversal of antagonistic techniques.

The Rood concept

Rood developed a treatment applicable to any neuromuscular dysfunction occurring at any age. It is based on normal sensorimotor learning and functions involved in the acquisition of co-ordinated movement. Her philosophy is concerned with the interaction of somatic, autonomic and psychic factors and their role in the regulation of motor behaviour. The overall framework of her approach is based on the concept that all functions can be related to one or two biological purposes.

1. *Mobility* — the survival of the individual through protection and mobility. Responses are rapid and either shield the individual or move him away from the stimulus;

2. *Stability* — the growth of the individual through pursuit and adaptation, which keeps him in contact with the environment.

The major concept is that neuromuscular mechanisms are characterised by dual functions that are complementary. Co-ordinated movement is the result of the introduction of mobilising and stabilising actions. As the relationship between these two actions develops, greater refinement of response is possible and there is effective control in direction and speed.

Rood identifies two major sequences in motor development distinctly different, yet inseparable:

1. Skeletal functions involving neck, trunk and extremities;
2. Vital functions involved in food intake and respiration.

According to Rood, the developmental sequence comprises the acquisition of four levels of function which she calls the ontogenetic motor patterns:

Level 1. Mobility. Movement is free and mobile only if it occurs in the full, normal excursion and has timing. Functional mobility occurs during the first three stages: withdrawal supine; roll over; pivot prone.

Level 2. Stability. Concerned with fixing the body to allow weight-bearing and also with dynamic holding during movement (pivot prone; co-contraction of the neck; elbow support; prone kneeling; static standing).

Level 3. Mobility superimposed on stability. If the individual is to function in a weight-bearing position he must have responses other than static maintenance of position.

Level 4. Skill. Refers to the co-ordinate movement rather than an exceptional degree of motor control.

Therapeutic procedures involve the application of stimuli to facilitate, inhibit or activate responses. The order of responses is important because the correct motor act results in feedback which may not only facilitate the correct response but may also provide sensory patterns of input for the succeeding patterns in the sequence (Stockmeyer 1967).

Various nerves and sensory receptors are described and classified into types: location; effect; response; distribution and indication. Techniques of stimulation are used to activate, facilitate or inhibit motor response. These include stroking, pressure, brushing, icing, heating, bone-pounding, muscle stretch, joint approximation, retraction and muscle pressure (Cash 1974).

Muscles are classified according to various physiological data, including their functional action. The appropriate stimuli for their actions are suggested. Stability muscles are first stimulated through high-threshold skin stimuli. High-threshold proprioceptive functions are stimulated by compression, stretch, resistance and pressure. Mobilising muscles are facilitated by quick stroking or quick application of ice.

In dealing with spasticity, Rood begins with fast brushing to the skin area over the stabiliser muscles followed by high-threshold stretch and joint approximation for inhibition of superficial muscles and facilitation of co-contraction of stabilisers. Mobility of proximal area can be achieved initially by heavy work patterns, especially those involving rotation at the joint needing an increase in range.

Only after inhibition of superficial holding and the activation of co-contraction by stabilisers are voluntary non-weight-bearing movements requested. Prior to this, voluntary effort usually reinforces the abnormal pattern because of the exaggerated effort that must go into working against the spastic pattern. Voluntary initiation should be preceded by appropriate inhibitory and facilitatory procedures so that it need not be difficult for the patient to achieve the response required (Stockmeyer 1967).

Use of EMG biofeedback

Opinions vary from pessimism to graded optimism as to the value of EMG biofeedback in the rehabilitation of stroke patients. No doubt, as with many other forms of treatment, biofeedback is another tool and a component of treatment, but not the strategy to be used for all disorders (Schwartz and Beatty 1977).

Baker *et al.* (1971) appear to have achieved promising results in alleviating both flaccid and spastic symptoms in stroke patients, regardless of the length of time since the cerebrovascular accident. The improvements in muscle function appear to be of lasting value since the patient leaves the clinical environment and is free of dependence upon feedback.

Instead of working to achieve a high EMG reading, the patient is working to attain silence and a nil meter reading. A joint is positioned so that the muscle is electrically silent; a limb is then carried passively through a range that stretches the spastic muscle. The patient is instructed to relax completely. Verbal reinforcement is given carefully and maintained throughout the session. Once control of spasticity through passive stretch has been learned, the patient is asked to contract the antagonistic muscle(s) whilst keeping the spastic muscle relaxed. A patient is thus helped to become aware of the feeling of 'tight' compared to 'relaxed' muscle.

The essential advantages of biofeedback are:

1. The corrective information is precise and applied continuously;
2. It may be used during an on-going activity such as walking;
3. Use of the device does not require of the patient sophisticated understanding of either electronics or their specific skill deficiencies. It is especially useful with older patients.

(Coudrey and Seeger 1981)

Conductive education

This form of care was developed by Professor Peto at the Institute for the Motor Disabled and Conductor College in Budapest. In common with other methods, Peto wanted to break up motor patterns, reduce spasticity and develop more selective movements. However, Peto relied on the patient's active participation and initiative rather than on the handling skill of the therapist. In conductive education, the patient learns a task that will lead to the acquisition of skills. Initially, he attempts the whole task observed by a 'conductor'. The task is then broken down into the appropriate task parts. As each task part is mastered, the intermediate steps are assimilated and new task parts introduced. It is believed that in this way the patients develop a wider repertoire of movement. The patient is taught how to guide his movements towards each task part of the total task by using his own speech (rhythmical intention).

Peto, by his definition of dysfunction, created a need for a new professional, the 'conductor', a person who co-ordinates the patient's day so that he may perform to his best ability intellectually, emotionally and physically. As with others involved in caring and rehabilitation, it is important that the conductor develops a singular personality — positive, dynamic and musical. The conductor's responsibilities may be identified:

1. To assess each patient; to observe each patient in normal life situations; to observe the patient in a group situation;
2. To organise and direct the timetable and day routine (including leisure time);

3. To initiate the patients into the group;
4. To direct the group;
5. To make up the task series;
6. To create a pleasant working atmosphere.

(after Cotton and Kinsman 1983)

Two conductors work with each group. All conductors have the same training and are equally knowledgeable about the patients, the timetables and the task series. The first conductor leads the group and initiates rhymthical intention. She decides if a task part has to be repeated or changed. The second conductor is there to assist the patients, which she does by moving from patient to patient anticipating their needs. She also helps in rhythmical intention and, if further repetition is needed, signals to the first conductor accordingly. Conductors may change roles during the day.

In conductive education, groupwork is the accepted format of work sessions. Patients work together in a group, which it is believed, stimulates, motivates and develops initiative. The conductor leads the group in a previously planned session. Within the group, the general attitude and bearing of each patient is noted in addition to his performance and disposition. The conductor selects the appropriate group for the patient. The patients in each group work together and identify with each other, sharing individual problems during rest and free periods. With the aid of rhythmical intention and through the conductor, the patient learns tasks or task parts and how to carry these over into the rest of the day. The patient is free to choose whether he works or not; this choice allows him to develop his own self-esteem and social awareness.

Groupwork may take place, at a table, in supine-lying, in free-sitting, in standing or in walking. Initially, the conductor uses a task series to observe the patient's ability within the group and completes an assessment of each patient. Using this information, the patient is allocated to the most suitable group (e.g. beginners, intermediate, advanced, or aphasic).

Summary

There are certain similarities between all the approaches described:

1. Involvement of the affected side in all aspects of treatment;
2. Attempts to relieve the effects of spasticity;

3. Attempts to re-educate specific patterns of normal movement;
4. Development of maximum functional activity bilaterally.

An atmosphere of rehabilitation

Successful rehabilitation requires that treatment and care must commence immediately after the onset of hemiplegia (Todd and Davies 1982). It is essential in the early stages to develop an atmosphere in which the patient will be motivated to learn to move again and which will enable him to be rehabilitated within the community. The importance of positioning the bed correctly whether at home or in the hospital is often not appreciated. Does there have to be a 'fixed' position for moveable ward furniture? A bed should be arranged so that the patient is made to look across to his affected side, reaching across the mid-line to get a glass of water or a tissue. It is this early motivation and education of sensory impairment that is so important and yet it is often neglected for the most unrealistic reasons.

It must be remembered that an homonymous hemianopia will result in disturbance of visual appreciation and that a patient may well have a limited field of vision and frequently a limited field of hearing. All rehabilitation should take place with the therapist within both visual and hearing fields.

Much has been written about the importance of positioning in terms of the head, shoulder and pelvic girdle: it is to be hoped that foot boards and hand splints have now been abandoned, as the problems they create are greater by far than any advantages they may have. A bed should not have a monkey pole and chain or overhead ring, but the patient should be encouraged to move himself about by pushing on his hands and feet, which is more natural than pulling up asymmetrically with one hand.

Relatives should be encouraged to attend the patient as frequently as possible and they must be reassured. They must have a clear explanation as to the importance of their role in the patient's recovery. Patients should be encouraged to dress in their own clothes as soon as they can. This helps motivation and demonstrates progress to both the patient and relatives.

Damage may be done to a patient's shoulder if the transfer from bed to chair is performed incorrectly. It is also frightening to the patient if the manoeuvre is performed without adequate explanation. The patient is assisted to the side of the bed and it is easier if the affected side is uppermost in side-lying. With one hand lifting the patient under the lying shoulder and the other hand pushing down on the uppermost pelvic bone, the patient is helped to sit up by shifting his weight and moving his head. Weight must be kept forwards at the hips. Normally, the patient will sit with his weight too far back and over onto the affected side; to counteract this tendency, practice is given in weight-transference. The physiotherapist should stand on the patient's affected side; fear of falling too often prevents a patient from mastering the art of weight-transference. It should be remembered that normally, when transferring weight forwards in the seated position, the head extends and when transferring weight backwards, it flexes. Similarly, when transferring weight to one side in the seated position, the head moves sideways in the opposite direction. Time must be allowed for adequate practice of balanced sitting. It is a waste of time to expect a patient either to stand or to walk until balanced sitting has been achieved. It is ridiculous to believe that it is morale-boosting to drag the patient around a room, supported between two persons.

In order to transfer a patient from bed to chair, the chair is placed at an angle to the bed on the affected side. The patient's arm rests gently on the therapist's shoulder in extension; the patient's feet are placed on the floor; the therapist's hand and arm should support the patient's shoulder and arm, particularly when the limb is hypotonic. The patient stands, bringing his pelvis and therefore his weight forwards — weight may then be transferred backwards by bending forwards at the hips when the patient may be asked to push his bottom back and sit down. If the patient does not have control of his pelvis, hip or knee, the therapist will have to protract the pelvis on the affected side and block the affected knee with her knees. If the pelvis is protracted sufficiently, the knee will not hyperextend. Transference should always be towards the affected side. In transference to the unaffected side, the patient will often extend the unaffected leg and 'push off' making the manoeuvre impossible and at the same time putting the therapist at risk from injury.

Throughout rehabilitation, compensation with the unaffected side is discouraged in order to allow the patient to develop movement which is as symmetrical as possible. At an early stage, correct weight-bearing provides good afferent stimulation and is most effective in normalising tone. In preparation for standing, some stability at the knee may be achieved by having the patient seated, extending his leg without either holding the knee or allowing it to hyperextend (spasticity may prevent this). With the knee straight, strong pressure is exerted through the heel in the direction of the hip. The patient then bends the knee slightly and straightens; this will help the patient to control his knee in the small range required for weight-bearing on the leg. In standing, weight-bearing on the affected leg is practised, for example, in stepping up and down to encourage the patient to take weight. It is essential that the pelvic girdle is protracted if a normal gait pattern is to be achieved and stairs managed safely. It is often the case that a patient can achieve success at individual movements, but finds it difficult and frustrating when attempting to put all parts into a total unified pattern.

Once the patient has sufficient tone and movement in his leg, walking can be assisted, provided that the therapist is able to prevent abnormal patterns of movement and a reasonable gait may be facilitated. If the patient is unable to weight-bear on the affected side, or unable to move his pelvis forwards, he will be unable to walk. Flexion at the hip and knee in preparation for heel-strike is related to the amount of extensor spasm in pelvis, hip and knee. Spasm may increase with the effort of walking and from the fear of falling; the therapist remains on the affected side at all times to minimise such fear.

Feeding is a necessary functional activity and one in which relatives may be of much assistance. Feeding is one of the best yet simplest ways of improving communication between the patient and relatives or therapist. It should be remembered that it is impossible to eat or speak if the tongue is held back and to the side; encouragement by wetting the lips or direct stimulation to the tongue is used to bring the tongue forwards. The patient should be seated and have the opportunity of eating 'solid' food. It is important that he has the food he likes and that foods with different textures should be offered to increase his awareness of what is in his mouth. Relatives are instructed to sit on the affected side of the patient or directly in front of him.

If the patient's lips do not close properly, brisk stroking of the affected side of his face in the direction of lip closure may be given. Should the patient drool or experience difficulty in swallowing, place a finger on the anterior one third of the tongue and push downwards and backwards. This will elevate the posterior one third of the tongue. Remove the finger, hold the jaw closed and ask the patient to swallow.

Prognosis

In the early days following a stroke, the emphasis is on whether the patient will survive or die. The mortality rate in the acute stage is high with 33 per cent of patients dying within three weeks: mortality increases with age. Adverse factors for survival include suppression of the level of consciousness (even drowsiness is a bad prognostic factor), failure to conjugate the gaze to the paralysed side and pulmonary changes.

Most recovery from stroke occurs within the first three months, but somewhere in the region of 10 per cent recovery occurs between three and twelve months. Community studies have shown that about 50 per cent of stroke survivors will achieve a full, or almost full, functional recovery (Langton Hewer 1984). Early development of spasticity in a limb is a good prognostic sign. The patient's prognosis is greatly influenced by the presence or absence of barriers to recovery outlined earlier in this chapter. However, it is important to give every patient a fair chance and not to dismiss those slow to respond too precipitantly. Adams (1974) found that it often took three or four months before the quality of survival could be predicted in many patients and it usually took another few months before it was possible to form an accurate assessment of the final outcome.

Community follow-up

Stroke rehabilitation is a continuous process and it should not stop when the patient is discharged from hospital. There is some evidence to suggest that long-term physiotherapy can prevent deterioration in some stroke survivors (Langton Hewer 1972). However, in general, the follow-up care of stroke patients leaves a lot to be desired. The frequency of psychological and social dysfunction following stroke tends to be underestimated. Because of the complex nature of the disability, the stroke victim needs a multidisciplinary approach not only whilst he is an in-patient, but, just as importantly, following his discharge. A number of support groups have developed in recent years, such as stroke clubs and the Stroke Volunteer Scheme. Each area should have a stroke programme to co-ordinate the overall approach to stroke care. In this way, patients are more likely to get maximum benefit from the statutory and voluntary agents involved in the field of stroke management (Lawrence and Christie 1979).

Following discharge, a patient may have physiotherapy as an out-patient in the physiotherapy department, or in the day hospital, or at home. Community physiotherapy and the day hospital are discussed later in the book, as are the various agencies that may be able to offer support, e.g. home help and meals-on-wheels (see Chapter 14).

Stroke clubs

Stroke clubs are organised by volunteers or voluntary bodies and their development in Britain has been encouraged by the Chest, Heart and Stroke Association. The club presents an opportunity for the stroke victim to get to know others who have experienced similar problems. It is also a regular social occasion and it may be the only such event in the lives of more severely affected patients who spend most of their time indoors. The stroke club also involves relatives and it gives them the opportunity to share experiences and to discuss problems.

The volunteer stroke scheme

The Volunteer Stroke Scheme was started by Valerie Eaton Griffith to help people with speech and communication problems after stroke. Its purpose is to encourage communication, however severe the loss of speech may be and to help overcome the resulting frustra-tion and apathy (Staunton 1984). Volunteers, in teams of two or three, go into each person's home on a regular weekly basis, spend-ing about one hour each with him or her. The volunteers aim to stimulate the stroke patient by drawing on their own and the patient's interests and hobbies. There is also a weekly club for the patients and outings are arranged to encourage self-confidence and to widen the patients' horizons once more.

REFERENCES

Adams, G.F. (1974) *Cerebrovascular disability and the ageing brain.* Churchill Livingstone, Edinburgh
Akhtar, A.J. and Garraway, W.M. (1982) 'Management of the elderly patient with stroke.' In F.I. Caird (ed), *Neurological disorders in the elderly*, Wright, Bristol

Amery, A., Birkenhager, W., Brixko, P. and Bulpitt, C. (1985) 'Mortality and morbidity results from the European working party on high blood pressure in the elderly trial.' *Lancet, 1*, 1349–54

Baker, M., Regenous, E., Wolf, S. and Basmajian, J.W. (1971) 'Developing strategies for biofeedback.' *Phys. Ther. 57*, 4

Basmajian, J.V., Regenous, E. and Baker, M. (1977) 'Rehabilitating stroke patients with biofeedback.' *Geriatrics, 7*, 24

Bobath, B. (1970) *Adult hemiplegia: evaluation and treatment*. Heinemann, London

Brocklehurst, J.C., Andrews, K., Morris, P., Richards, B.R. and Laycock, P.L. (1978) 'Why admit stroke patients to hospital?' *Age and ageing, 7, 2*, 100

Brunnstrom, S. (1970) *Movement therapy in hemiplegia*. Harper and Row, New York

Carr, J.H. and Shepherd, R.B. (1979) *Early care of the stroke patient: a positive approach*. William Heinemann Medical Books, London

Cash, J. (1974) *Neurology for physiotherapists*. Faber and Faber, London

Cotton, E. and Kinsman, R. (1983) *Conductive education for adult hemiplegia*. Churchill Livingstone, Edinburgh

Coudrey, D. and Seeger, B. (1981) 'Biofeedback devices as an adjunct to physiotherapy.' *Physiotherapy, 67, 12*, 371–6

Evans, J.G. and Caird, F.I. (1982) 'Epidemiology of neurological disorders.' In F.I. Caird (ed), *Neurological disorders in the elderly*, Wright, Bristol

Hughes, E. (1972) 'Bobath and Brunnstrom — comparison of two methods of treatment of a left hemiplegic.' *Physiotherapy Canada, 24*, 5–11

Johnstone, M. (1976) *The stroke patient — principles of rehabilitation*. Churchill Livingstone, Edinburgh

Knott, M. and Voss, D. (1977) *Proprioceptive neuromuscular facilitation*. Harper and Row, New York

Langton-Hewer, R. (1972) 'Stroke Units.' *Brit. Med. J., 1*, 52

——— (1984) 'Recovery from stroke.' In J. Grimley-Evans and F.I. Caird (eds), *Advanced Geriatric Medicine*, Pitman, London

Lawrence, L. and Christie, D. (1979) 'Quality of life after stroke. a three year follow-up.' *Age and Ageing, 8*, 167–72

McCarthy, S.T., Turner, J.J., Roberston, D., Hawkey, C.J. and Macey, D.J. (1977) 'Low-dose heparin as a prophylaxis against deep-vein thrombosis after acute stroke.' *Lancet, 2*, 800–1

Schwartz, G.F. and Beatty, J. (1977) 'Biofeedback Theory and Research.' *Academic Papers*

Staunton, E. (1984) 'The volunteer stroke scheme.' In B. Isaacs and H. Evers (eds), *Innovations in the care of the elderly*, Croom Helm, London

Stockmeyer, S. (1967) 'An interpretation of the approach of Rood in the treatment of neuromuscular dysfunction.' *Am. J. Phys. Med., 46*, 1–9

Todd, J.M. and Davies, P.M. (1982) 'Hemiplegia — 2.' In P.A. Downie (ed), *Cash's textbook of neurology for physiotherapists*, 3rd edn, Faber and Faber, London

Voss, D. (1967) 'Proprioceptive neuromuscular facilitation.' *Am. J. Phys. Med., 46*, 10

Warlow, E. (1978) 'Venous thrombo-embolism after stroke.' *Am. Heart J. 96 (3)*, 283–5

6

Treatment of Musculo-skeletal Disorders

Musculo-skeletal disorders are common in elderly people. Most older people have degenerative changes in their joints, tendons and muscles. Bone loss is part of normal ageing. Bone deposition increases rapidly during the first 17 years of life (the period of growth) and continues to increase more gradually for about another 12 years. After the age of 45 there is a gradual loss of bone and this is more marked in women (Exton-Smith 1983). People with denser bones at maturity are less likely to develop problems with the gradual loss of bone during ageing than those who have low bone density at maturity. It should be remembered that many of those who survive into advanced old age are among the biological elite and some individuals aged 80 have more bone than others at the age of 30 (Exton-Smith and Overstall 1979).

Muscular strength declines with age and this decline is usually associated with a parallel decrease in the bone density. The predicted grip of the right hand in the male decreases from 44.0 kg (97 lb) at 60 to 32.1 kg (71 lb) at 89. There is also a decrease in the ratio of muscle tissue to fatty tissue in the body as the individual ages.

OSTEOARTHROSIS

The most obvious feature of osteoarthrosis is that it increases in frequency with age. This does not mean that it is an expression of senescence; it simply shows that osteoarthrosis takes many years to develop.

Apley (1976) distinguishes between two types of cartilage degeneration:

1. Limited cartilage loss, seen mainly away from load-bearing areas, probably due to 'wear and tear';
2. Progressive cartilage destruction, which is always maximal in the major load-bearing areas and is associated with symptomatic osteoarthrosis.

There is no single cause of osteoarthrosis; it results from a disparity between the stress applied to articular cartilage and the ability of the cartilage to withstand stress. Factors implicated in aetiology include previous joint disease or trauma, sex ratio, age of onset, relation to menopause and hereditary factors. A typical feature of osteoarthrosis is its intermittent course, with periods of symptomatic remission. Sometimes, it is noted that as the joint becomes stiffer, it becomes less painful.

Symptoms

Pain is the usual presenting symptom. Often it is worse on rising from bed and again at the end of a day's activity. It is aggravated by extremes of movement or by unaccustomed exertion. Early on, it is relieved by rest, but with time, relief comes more slowly and is less complete. The worst pain often occurs in bed at night, when the patient finds it difficult to find a position that is comfortable. Helal (1965) demonstrated three sources of pain: capsular (on extreme of range); muscular (on movement); and venous (at rest).

Stiffness is common at first after periods of rest and later becomes constant and progressive. Swelling in peripheral joints may be due to an effusion, to synovial and capsular thickening or to osteophytes. Deformity often precedes the onset of osteoarthrosis, but may result from muscle imbalance, capsular contracture or joint instability.

Signs

The pattern of involvement is variable. The patient generally complains of one or two joints, though examination may reveal greater involvement. Swelling and deformity may be obvious in peripheral joints; at the hip deformity is often masked by postural adjustments in the pelvis and spine, but may be checked by Thomas' test. In long-standing cases, muscle atrophy may be apparent and local tenderness is common. Movement is always restricted, yet may be painless within a restricted range; extension, abduction and medial rotation are normally limited. There may be crepitus accompanying the movement. In later stages, instability may occur.

Treatment principles

Treatment may be divided into early, intermediate and late stages.

Early

The aims are:

1. To relieve pain;
2. To prevent further strain or trauma on an affected joint;
3. To improve muscle power and maintain mobility;
4. To improve nutrition of the cartilage by restoration of physiological movement.

(after Hyde 1980)

Analgesics and anti-inflammatory agents can control pain for many years. However, over-medication should be avoided; it may lead to 'analgesic degeneration'. Conservative methods include short-wave diathermy (pulsed) (Wagstaff, Wagstaff and Downey 1986), infra-red, interferential, Therafield and so on: the main choice being dependent upon the area(s) most affected. Clarke *et al.* (1974) showed that ice was the most beneficial method of giving short-term relief of pain in osteoarthrosis.

It is important to maintain and improve muscle strength as the disease process will lead to an increasing instability in affected joints. Consideration must be given to the position in which exercise is performed and the range through which movement will take place. For example, in giving quadriceps work, some believe that an attempt should be made to align the tibia and the femur so that vastus medialis may be contracted in its inner range with the therapist placing one hand on the medial side of the knee joint and the other hand on the lateral side of the calf. Excessive range may tend to increase trauma to a joint and inappropriate activity encourage deformity. When pain is predominant, isometric rather than isotonic muscle work is preferred. Hold–relax may be used to attempt to increase range. Peripheral joint mobilisations may increase range by reducing capsular strain and thereby pain (Maitland 1977).

Common-sense measures to reduce load include weight loss, the use of walking aids, avoidance of unnecessary stress (climbing stairs) and even intermittent periods of complete rest. Attention to footwear is important.

It is crucial that a patient has the disease carefully explained to him in the early stages and that he is reassured that though it will impose limitation on activity, it is not crippling. Many patients believe that arthritis, rheumatism, etc. are all the same and they will frequently know of friends who are severely disabled. Patients are perturbed at the prospect of the change in appearance that deformity brings about (Goffman 1968). It should be emphasised that treatment and support given by family and friends is essential: patients often feel concern over the burden on the family that their impaired mobility may bring (Wright and Owen 1976).

Self-care. Adler (1985) has described the importance of early emphasis on self-care. The patient should be given advice on the careful use of joints, for example, the correct use of walking aids reduces the compressive forces applied to a joint. Careful explanation is often needed to persuade the patient to use a walking stick to preserve his joint, help decrease pain and increase function. Preservation is an important concept for the patient to grasp if he is to adapt his activities to reduce strain on the joint. The patient must be shown exercises to increase muscle strength and how to perform these at home. As pain is the symptom that brings a patient to the hospital, he may be shown how to apply ice to the knee joint for example, using a bag of frozen peas, the skin being protected with a paper towel or wet flannel.

Intermediate

If signs and symptoms increase, then at some joints (chiefly the hip and knee) realignment osteotomy is indicated (Apley 1976), or arthroplasty. Such operative techniques should be performed while the joint is still stable and mobile. Pain relief is often dramatic.

Late

Progressive joint destruction with increasing pain, disability and deformity usually require reconstructive surgery. Arthrodesis may be the surgery of choice if (a) stiffness is acceptable and (b) neighbouring joints are not likely to be prejudiced. With arthroplasty, timing is essential (Apley 1976), too early and the odds against a durable result lengthen in proportion to the demands of activity: too late and bone destruction, deformity, stiffness and muscle atrophy make the operation more difficult and the results more unpredictable.

RHEUMATOID ARTHRITIS

Rheumatoid arthritis is a systemic disorder, chronic in nature, which involves mainly peripheral joints. The joint damage occurs as a consequence of proliferation and inflammation of the synovial membrane, which leads to erosion of the articular cartilage and gradual destruction of the supporting structures.

In the elderly, rheumatoid arthritis is usually long-established, with the inflammation that has largely subsided leaving varying degrees of deformity and permanent damage. However, its onset may occur in patients over seventy and eighty and may be explosive, with more systemic upset and widespread muscle pain than is usual in younger patients (Brewerton 1979).

There is an increase in incidence of rheumatoid arthritis among persons who are 60 and older and this has a substantial socio-economic impact on society as a result of the progressive physical impairment the disease brings about (Meenan, Yelin and Nevitt 1981). Rheumatoid arthritis has no typical course. In most cases it evolves slowly, but it can develop abruptly and progress rapidly. The shoulders are often affected in patients over the age of 60. Older patients tend to get more severe disease and age has been found to correlate significantly with clinical outcome. Anger, intolerance and apathy make treatment difficult, as patients can be unco-operative and can resent assistance (Slannka 1980). It is not necessarily an exacerbation if an elderly patient with long-established rheumatoid arthritis deteriorates and it is wise to think of alternative serious possibilities (e.g. subluxation of the cervical spine; supurative arthritis; spontaneous fractures due to osteoporosis).

The practical management and care of rheumatoid arthritis is difficult and complex. A knowledge of all potential deformities and deforming factors is needed. In the elderly, there are frequently multiple deformities with severe destructive changes, especially in the weight-bearing joints. The struggle is to keep the patient on his feet with some degree of independence. Care of the rheumatoid patient demands a team approach. Although the number of joints and the extent to which they are affected will vary according to the stage of the disease, the patient must be treated with an holistic approach.

Deformities

In the hand

There may be ulnar deviation at the metacarpophalangeal joints. Swan neck deformity of the fingers may be seen. This arises from hyperextension of the proximal interphalangeal joint with fixed flexion of the distal interphalangeal joint. Boutonnière deformity may also occur — the proximal interphalangeal joint protrudes through the extensor expansion, the two halves of which slip forward until attempts to extend the joint produce flexion at this joint but extension at the distal interphalangeal joint.

In the wrist

Early erosive changes in the ulnar styloid and, later, cystic changes in the distal ends of both radius and ulna, lead to a position of palmar flexion and deviation.

In the feet

Subluxation of the metatarsophalangeal joints, with the toes displaced upwards and fixed flexion at the interphalangeal joint, results in dropped metatarsal heads; these then become weight-bearing.

In the cervical spine

The problem is not so much deformity, but of instability with subluxation at the atlanto-axial joint.

In the hip

Flexion deformity with lateral rotation may be present.

In the knees

Flexion deformity with varus or valgus components may be present.

Rheumatoid arthritis cannot be cured by drugs, but there are a number of agents that dampen the inflammatory process and thus impede structural damage. The most commonly used agents are anti-inflammatory drugs such as salicylates and related compounds. More toxic agents include gold, hydroxychloroquine, penicillamine and immunosuppressive agents such as azathiaprine. Low-dose steroid therapy is also used. Myopathy, bone loss and fluid retention are a few of the many side effects associated with these drugs. Therefore, the more that can be done without drugs in this condition, the better.

Because of the systemic manifestations of the disease and the pain which is at times severe and unremitting, rest is essential. However, for the older patient, total immobility is a real danger and it must be explained to the patient that 'taking completely to bed' is not wise. One must strike the appropriate balance between activity and rest and this will be determined by the level of disease activity and other pathology present.

Much controversy surrounds the appropriate degree of rest suitable for a patient and a general consensus would tend to favour local immobilisation with or without isometric activity to the affected joints. Partridge and Duthie (1969) report beneficial effects from immobilisation.

Hyde (1980) suggests that the role of the physiotherapist in rheumatoid arthritis is:

1. To assess and re-assess patients;
2. To monitor patients' progress;
3. To offer advice on the indication for physiotherapy and the most appropriate form of treatment;
4. To review and revise home programmes;
5. To review and adjust splints and appliances.

She considers that out-patient attendance as opposed to home care is only indicated when:

1. The patient has just been diagnosed (less likely in the elderly);
2. There has been rapid or marked deterioration;
3. There is a specific objective.

Criteria for admission and in-patient care might be:

1. Where there are multitudinous and complex problems to be reviewed or where the patient's condition has deteriorated rapidly;
2. Social reasons.

It is essential that the physiotherapist involves the patient's relatives in the management regime. It is particularly important that relatives understand clearly the purpose of the activity programme and rest periods and of the balance between them. When there is loss of function, it is in part the role of the physiotherapist to find alternative ways of accomplishing the activity; for this, the therapist must be familiar with the patient's home environment.

Regimes of exercise need to be constantly revised to take account of improvement or progression of the disease, as well as to help motivate and encourage the patient. One of the risks of a home regime of 'do-it-yourself' therapy is that a motivated or over-enthusiastic relative will push too far and increase the irritability of joints and so create more pain. Thus any instruction must be specific and vague terms are to be avoided.

In order to strengthen muscle power, maximum resistance is necessary. In the rheumatoid patient, this is the resistance that will permit a smooth, co-ordinated contraction in all parts of the range. This avoids strain on an affected joint. Joints should be put through a daily regime of full-range activity. It is not enough for a patient simply to 'be active' during the day. Active rather than passive movements are to be encouraged; this will avoid the overzealous going beyond an accepted range of movement.

In order to relieve the tension over swollen joint capsules and the associated irritable synovial linings, patients adopt characteristic deformities. The deformities create a lengthening of structure on one side and shortening on the opposite side, with resultant muscle atrophy and muscle imbalance. Ultimately, there is a total upset in body mechanics, leading to bizarre joint and movement patterns. Such deformity is minimised by patient education, exercise, passive stretching and splinting. Care should be taken in order to avoid overstretching, especially if ligaments are lax.

Frequently, in the older patient, there is loss of muscle power, loss of mobility and pain, all of which create distress for the patient and relatives. It is in the maintenance of function that close liaison between the physiotherapist and occupational therapist is needed. Ekblom *et al.* (1975) have shown improvement in function following periods of physiotherapy in stages of articular cartilage involvement and in stages of destruction of joint surfaces. Nordemar *et al.* (1976) have demonstrated the importance of effective regimes of home care.

Patients are frequently referred for physiotherapy for the relief of pain. Heat, hot packs, short-wave diathermy, wax baths, interferential and diadynamic currents have all been tried with varying degrees of success.

Table 6.1: Assessment of activities of daily living in the rheumatoid patient

Pouring boiling liquids Beating, mixing by hand Cutting bread Opening tins Carrying trays	} A	Into bath Out of bath Kneeling Carrying bucket Stairs Cleaning windows Opening windows	} B	
Getting onto toilet Sitting up to table Getting off toilet Getting in/out of bed	} C	Door handles Winding watch	} D	
Cutting meat Buttering bread Using knife, fork, spoon	} E	Writing Matches	} F	
Wringing Washing hands/nails Washing face	} G			

A = upper limb and shoulder
B = whole body
C = hip and knee primarily
D, E, F, and G = different uses of arm, wrist and hand

Source: Badley, Lee and Wood 1979

The physiotherapist must not be put off by the apparently difficult patient. It must be remembered that the effect of the disease may be devastating. It may have necessitated early retirement; 85 per cent of patients need to alter their leisure-time activities and 18 per cent will have had to change their residence.

Badley, Lee and Wood (1979) have devised a valuable means of assessment of activities of daily living in the rheumatoid patient, which relates loss of function and areas of loss of mobility (*see* Table 6.1).

GOUT

High levels of uric acid in the blood predispose to the development of gout. Thiazide diuretics, polycythaemia and renal disease are among the factors that precipitate the condition in the elderly. Usually gout involves one joint, the metatarsophalangeal joint being

91

the most favoured, but it can affect any joint. The joint becomes red, swollen and extremely painful. The pain results from the deposition of urate crystals between the articular surfaces and repeated attacks may lead to chronic changes in the joints. Crystals may also be deposited in the skin and in the cartilage of the ear and nose where they are known as tophi; the olecranon bursa is a common site for tophi.

The acute attack responds to anti-inflammatory drugs such as indomethacin or, alternatively, colchicine. Allopurinol may be used to reduce the level of uric acid in the blood on a long-term basis.

PSEUDOGOUT — PYROPHOSPHATE ARTHROPATHY

In this condition, pyrophosphate crystals are deposited in the joints, but unlike gout, there is a predilection for larger joints such as the knee. Lines of calcification are seen in the fibrocartilage or synovial membrane of joints (chondrocalcinosis) and pyrophosphate crystals will be found on examination of a synovial fluid aspirate. Treatment during the acute stage is with anti-inflammatory drugs. Chondro-calcinosis is not always associated with pyrophosphate arthropathy.

PAGET'S DISEASE

This disease of old age affects about six per cent of the population aged over 70. In Paget's disease, both formation and resorption of bone are abnormal, with the result that thicker, poor quality bone is laid down in an unco-ordinated manner. The bone, although more bulky than normal bone, is weak from a structural point of view. Any bone can be affected but the pelvis, tibia and skull are frequently involved. Usually the patients are asymptomatic and the condition is diagnosed when the patient is x-rayed for another condi-tion. Big head, bent back and bow legs is a classical description for patients with marked skeletal involvement. The patient may complain of bone pain and fractures occur particularly in the shaft of the femur. Neurological problems like deafness may develop if the enlarged bone compresses a nerve.

Investigation

The serum alkaline phosphatase is high and x-rays show character-istic thickening with destruction of normal bone patterns. Most patients do not need treatment. Those that need therapy may be started on the hormone calcitonin and, more recently, diphosphon-ates have also been used in treatment.

OSTEOPOROSIS

In osteoporosis, the amount of bone per unit volume is diminished, but the remaining bone is normal in quality. Although the actual size of the bones is unchanged, the amount of bone tissue is reduced. The aetiology is still unknown but it is thought to be due to increased resorption of bone. As pointed out earlier in the chapter, the density of bone at maturity will be a major factor in determining whether the amount of bone in an individual over the years will be sufficient to cause osteoporosis. Bone resorption is accelerated in women during the first ten years after menopause and this is thought to be due to the fall in oestrogen levels. Calcium deficiency may be a factor and vitamin D deficiency may be particularly important in the genesis of osteoporosis in the elderly. The malabsorption of calcium found in patients with fractures of the femoral neck is almost certainly due to vitamin D deficiency. Immobility may also lead to osteoporosis either localised after a fracture or hemiplegia, or generalised in elderly patients who sit about all day. Long-term steroid therapy also leads to osteoporosis. Most patients with osteoporosis have no symptoms. It may be detected when a patient is x-rayed for some other condi-tion. About 25 per cent of elderly patients have demonstrable reduc-tion in bone density (Chalmers 1980). The patient frequently presents for the first time with a fracture. Fracture of the vertebral body with severe back pain is a common presentation. Many of the patients develop a deformity known as Dowager's Hump because of wedging of the mid-thoracic vertebrae.

Bone biochemistry is normal in osteoporosis and the diagnosis is usually made on the basis of clinical presentation and radiology. There is an increased translucency which affects all bones, but particularly trabecular bone. Changes are most obvious in the vertebral bodies which, as the disease progresses usually become distorted in shape with some collapsing completely.

The treatment of osteoporosis is very controversial. Oestrogen therapy and calcium supplements are used to prevent the accelerated bone loss after the menopause. Elderly patients with established osteoporosis may be treated with calcium and low-dose vitamin D supplements. Fluoride and androgenic steroids are also advocated by some workers as therapy for osteoporosis.

OSTEOMALACIA

Osteomalacia is caused by vitamin D deficiency. The characteristic feature of the disease is deficient calcification of the bone matrix with the result that there is an increased amount of non-calcified matrix known as osteoid around the bone trabeculae. In osteo-malacia, it is the quality of the bone which alters rather than the quantity as in osteoporosis. As well as the bone changes, osteo-malacia also produces muscle stiffness and weakness. Vitamin D is a fat-soluble vitamin present in foods such as dairy products and fish and it is also synthesised in the skin on exposure to sunlight. Old people are particularly likely to become deficient in vitamin D as their diet is often inadequate and they may not be able to obtain suffi-cient exposure to sunlight. Patients with malabsorption, or with renal and liver disease are also more likely to develop osteomalacia.

Osteomalacia has an insidious onset. Generalised pain is an important clinical feature, but it should not be forgotten that muscle weakness may often be striking. The weakness usually affects the proximal muscles and the patient may experience difficulty in getting up from a chair or in climbing stairs. Marked weakness will lead to the characteristic 'waddling gait'. The patient develops difficulty in lifting his feet when walking and the pelvis is tilted as a compensatory movement. Those with shoulder muscle weakness may notice difficulty in washing their face or combing their hair. Deformities such as kyphoscoliosis are common.

If it remains undiagnosed, pain may become very severe and the patient may find even the weight of the bed clothes intolerable. Vitamin D deficiency is thought to be an important factor in the aetiology of fractured femur in the elderly. A study at Leeds showed that 20 to 30 per cent of women and about 40 per cent of men with femoral neck fracture had evidence of osteomalacia on bone biopsy (Aaron *et al.* 1974). However, subsequent studies would indicate this to be a high figure. Lower ribs are also a common site for fracture.

Blood tests show a raised serum alkaline phosphatase. Serum calcium may be normal or low and inorganic phosphorous is low.

The serum alkaline phosphatase is most clearly related to the bone changes. Vitamin D levels can now be measured in the blood. X-rays will show diminished bone density. In advanced cases, the bones are deformed and pseudo-fractures (looser zones), which are bands of rarefaction, can be seen along the border of the scapula, pubic rami, ribs, neck of humerus and femur. Bone biopsy will confirm diagnosis.

The condition is treated with vitamin D and calcium supplements. The underlying cause of the initial deficiency (e.g. dietary mal-absorption or lack of sunshine) must be tackled. Preventive measures should also be taken so that at-risk patients such as those who are socially isolated or immobile do not develop the condition. Providing adequate social support may be sufficient but there may be also a need for increasing the vitamin D content of the diet (e.g. more milk) or by giving vitamin D supplements. Two halibut oil tablets daily would be sufficient.

POLYMYALGIA RHEUMATICA

Polymyalgia rheumatica is a disease which affects older people (Apley 1982). It is related to temporal or giant-cell arteritis, which is caused by an inflammatory process in the arteries. The exact pathology is still a matter of debate. Its clinical onset is usually sudden and the patient develops stiffness and pain of the proximal limb muscles (usually the upper limbs). The involved muscles may be tender to touch. Because of the stiffness, the patient may have difficulty in getting out of bed or out of a chair and he may have difficulty in washing and performing other daily tasks. The erythro-cyte sedimentation rate is elevated and there is a dramatic response to treatment with steroids.

PROGRESSIVE SYSTEMIC SCLEROSIS (SCLERODERMA)

The most characteristic features of the disease is the taut and thickened skin which gives rise to the name scleroderma. The basic aetiology is unknown, but fibrosis of the skin and internal organs results from over-production of collagen. It is more common in women and there is often a history of Raynaud's syndrome. The disease may be a progressive one from earlier adult life into old age, but it often begins in the elderly and in this age group, the condition

95

is usually benign (Hodkinson 1971). Physiotherapy does not produce dramatic results. However, attempts should be made to minimise contractures and the loss of mobility and to preserve muscle power as long as possible.

POLYMYOSITIS

Polymyositis is a disease that is seen mainly in older adults. It is rare and the basic pathology is an inflammatory myopathy of unknown aetiology. The main feature is a characteristic rash involving the eyelids, cheeks and the exposed areas. The condition is treated with high-dose steroids. There is an increased association with malignancy and the disease has a particularly poor prognosis in the elderly.

SYSTEMIC LUPUS ERYTHEMATOSUS

This connective-tissue disease occurs primarily in younger women but it can also occur in the elderly. The disease is associated with the production of a large number of antibodies to the patient's own tissues. It usually has an insidious onset in the elderly with fatigue, weight loss and polyarthritis; the patient may become very immobile. The condition has a better long-term prognosis in the elderly. Drugs used in the treatment include, anti-inflammatory agents, hydroxychloroquine and steroids. Systemic lupus erythematosus (SLE) can be induced by drugs such as procainamide and hydrallazine and this is more likely to occur in the older patient.

SHOULDER–HAND SYNDROME

The occurrence of a group of conditions causing vasomotor and dystrophic changes of the shoulder and hand is well recognised. The variety of apparent causes and the variable manifestations led to a wide range of names being applied to the condition now known as 'Shoulder–hand syndrome'. Steinbrocher and Argyros (1958) found that 26 per cent followed cardiac infarction, 10 per cent were post-traumatic, 6 per cent post hemiplegic, 20 per cent associated with cervical degenerative changes and the remainder idiopathic.

It seems that both sexes are affected equally and there is a prodromal stage between the painful causative insult (if any) and the onset of the syndrome. The first phase is that of a painful shoulder with a persistent ache being exaggerated by movement. The patient finds it hard to sleep. Restriction of movement is in a capsular pattern, though the restricted movement is relatively pain-free. Pain spreads from the shoulder to the hand and vasomotor changes ensue. There is swelling, colour change, sweating and stiffening of the fingers. The second stage sees atrophy of the shoulder muscles and dystrophic and nail changes in the hand, but normally with lessening of pain and disability. The syndrome may be unilateral, bilateral, partial or complete, but curiously, it seldom affects the elbow.

There is debate as to the place and value of physiotherapy in this condition. Cuddigan and Mathews (1971) believe that supervision of active and assisted exercise appropriate to the general condition of a patient with myocardial infarction or cerebrovascular accident may avert the syndrome in the prodromal stage.

In the first stage of the syndrome, reassurance is perhaps the key element. The patient can be told that the condition is self-limiting and that the situation is reversible. The primary aim is to relieve pain. There may be contraindications to using cold therapy, however interferential 90–100 Hz or 100–32 Hz, or Therafield with antennae placed locally and a frequency of 80 Hz may be helpful. Treatment of the hand is aimed at maintenance of movement. Gentle passive stretching of the fingers is attempted, but force and the production of pain must be avoided for fear of providing further afferent stimulation and reflex activity. Once pain has subsided in the shoulder and the patient finds sleep less disturbed, gentle mobilisations may be attempted and pulsed short-wave diathermy may be given.

When the condition has been recognised and treated at an early stage, gradual progressive improvement without lasting sequelae is to be expected. Many months may pass before complete resolution.

SHOULDER PAIN

Various disorders may trigger a vascular response in the cuff. Degenerative changes in the tendons of the rotator cuff are common (Brewerton 1979). In the older patient, rotator-cuff symptoms tend to be more persistent than in younger age groups.

In chronic tendinitis (painful arc syndrome), the patient complains of pain in the shoulder and over the deltoid muscle. Often the pain is worse at night and may be severe on attempting activities such as dressing. The shoulder looks normal, but is tender along the edge of the acromion and anteriorly in the space between the acromion and coracoid process. On abduction, pain is aggravated between 60° and 120°. Kessel and Watson (1977) have pointed out that in one-third of patients, the lesion is in the posterior part of the cuff, in one-third it is anterior (subscapularis) and in the remaining third, it is the supraspinatus. If treatment is to be effective, it is essential to identify the site of the lesion. Careful palpation and passive movement of the shoulder with the arm in varying degrees of rotation may pinpoint the tender spot, or alternatively, the use of Flexitherm or combined ultrasound and interferential or diadynamic may give a more accurate result (Wadsworth and Chanmugam 1983). Osteoarthrosis of the acromioclavicular joint is not uncommon: the joint feels thick and is tender to touch, abduction is painful during the final 60° and adduction in horizontal flexion is very painful.

The treatment for all these conditions is transverse frictions. However, it is essential to locate the area accurately and to apply frictions in an adequate manner.

Adhesive capsulitis (frozen shoulder) probably starts in the same way as chronic tendinitis, but spreads to involve the entire tendinous cuff, which becomes thick, vascular and infiltrated with lymphocytes and plasma cells; it sticks to the humeral head and the infra-articular 'gusset' of the capsule. The result is a capsular pattern of limitation, with lateral rotation, the most-affected movement and flexion, the least-affected movement. Pain is felt at the deltoid insertion and radiates along the outer side of the arm.

There are three phases of disability, each lasting three to eight months:

1. Increasing pain and increasing stiffness;
2. Decreasing pain with persistent stiffness;
3. Painless return of movement.

In the first phase, the aims of treatment are:

1. To give the patient reassurance;
2. To relieve pain;
3. To prevent further suffering while recovery is awaited.

Pain may be resolved by heat or cold, by high- and medium-frequency modalities such as Therafield, interferential and ultra-

Reiz, or by laser. Active exercise tends to be too painful. However, accessory movements may be given although antero-posterior glide is avoided as pressure on the gleno-humeral ligaments frequently causes pain. As pain subsides, sling suspension may be started together with pendular exercises. The patient is advised that moderation and regularity is to be preferred to sporadic, vigorous activity. Once pain has subsided, active exercise is given with the emphasis on function and day-to-day activities.

FOOT PROBLEMS

Of the entire musculo-skeletal system, the foot is perhaps the foremost in showing the ravages of time, abetted by the static stresses imposed by weight-bearing and shoes (Jahss 1979). Treatment tends to be palliative, falling into the realm of mechanotherapy: special shoes, shoe corrections, protective padding and arch supports.

Protective padding should be applied specifically for each individual patient. To provide a support from 'off the shelf' can only provide relief of pain on a chance basis. Padding consists of moleskin and adhesive-backed piano felt or sponge rubber. Plastazote and other materials now on the market have the advantage of more accurate moulding. More permanent forms of relief consist of corrections permanently fitted into a shoe or removable insoles. In cases of severe foot deformity, commercial orthopaedic shoes and custom-made shoes may be required. The most common skin lesions in the elderly are painful calluses and ulcers due to impaired vascular supply.

It must be remembered that an elderly person may be unable to bend over in order to cut his nails; the nails themselves may be too hard to cut. A chiropodist is required to visit the patient regularly to clip the nails or to grind them.

HALLUX VALGUS AND ASSOCIATED SPLAY FOOT

Whereas in the younger patient the deformity may be surgically corrected, in the elderly this may not be possible and conservative treatment remains the method of choice. All patients with hallux valgus can be made more comfortable by careful attention to footwear. Shoes should be wide-fitting and the uppers soft. Padding may be incorporated to protect the bunion. The patient should be shown a programme of foot exercises, avoiding activity that will encourage activity of the long flexors, but concentrating on intrinsic muscle work; activity such as 'rolling up a bandage with the toes' or 'picking up objects with the toes' must be avoided. In order to assist the patient to feel the correct movement, a Faradic foot bath may be used or appropriate interferential frequency. One pad is placed under the forefoot and a small disc electrode is used to locate the motor point of abductor hallucis muscle; this point is variable and found on the medial side of the foot by 'trial and error'. The intrinsic muscles may be worked as a group by placing one pad under the heel and placing a second pad diagonally under the metatarsal heads. The re-education programme consists of five stages:

1. The patient observes and feels the contraction and subsequent movement;
2. The patient works with the machine to produce the correct movement;
3. The patient holds the contraction during a relaxation phase;
4. The patient gains the contraction, with the machine providing progressively less and less assistance;
5. The patient gains the contraction without the assistance of the machine.

HALLUX RIGIDUS

The rigidity is due to degenerative arthritis. In contrast to hallux valgus, males are more commonly affected. The patient experiences pain on walking, especially on slopes or on rough ground. There is often a callosity under the medial side of the distal phalanx. On assessment, it is noted that the outer side of the sole of the shoe may be unduly worn — the result of rolling the foot outwards to avoid pressure on the big toe. The metatarsophalangeal joint feels enlarged and tender. Dorsiflexion is restricted and painful. A quarter-inch sole-rocker may abolish pain by allowing the foot to roll without the necessity for dorsiflexion at the metatarsophalangeal joint.

HAMMER TOES

The proximal toe joint is fixed in flexion, while the distal joint and the metatarsophalangeal joints are extended. The second toe is commonly affected. Shoe pressure may produce painful corns or callosities on the dorsum of the toes and under the prominent metatarsal head.

Hammer-toe shields are made depending on whether the hammering is flexible or rigid. The flexible pad consists of a thick half-moon-shaped piece of felt or sponge placed proximal to the dorsal corn; on the plantar surface, a plug of felt is placed just under the middle phalanx with the proximal portion tapered in a wedge. The shield is secured with strips of adhesive. In rigid hammer toes, a full oval protective shield is placed with a hole for the dorsal corn; on the plantar surface, a plug of felt is cut to fit into the hollow.

METATARSALGIA

Metatarsalgia would seem to be a greater problem in women than in men, possibly because wearers of shoes with lower heels are less likely to develop such symptoms. The patient and his shoes need to be methodically assessed.

The conservative treatment of metatarsalgia consists of a mechanical means of relieving pressure. Mild cases may be relieved with a one-eighth inch insole. A metatarsal pad needs to be fitted to each individual patient in such a way that it fits just proximal to the second, third and fourth metatarsal heads. Often there is too little weight-bearing on the first and fifth metatarsal heads and, in such cases, in addition to the metatarsal pad, insole raises are required to distribute weight more evenly. Heel height should be the minimum a patient can comfortably wear.

CALCANEAL SPUR

The pain is often bilateral and most severe on initiation of weight-bearing. Conservative treatment consists of cutting a well from the inside of the heel of the shoe under the painful area; the well is filled with sponge rubber and the entire heel covered with about three-eighths of an inch of firm foam rubber. This produces a soft but resilient shallow cup into which the heel sinks. Ultrasound therapy (pulsed 1:4; 3 MHz; 1.5 Wcm^2) may be tried over the painful area or laser for three minutes.

FRACTURES

The likelihood of an individual fracturing a bone rises with increasing age. Post-menopausal women are at increased risk of fracturing the distal radius (Colles' fracture) and as they grow older, vertebral and femoral fractures become more common. The risk of fracture is so great that 25 per cent of women who survive into old age will have suffered at least one fracture by the age of 80. Older people not only have brittle bones but they are at higher risk of falling than younger people for a variety of reasons (see p. 105). Despite the high risk, fractures are constantly missed in the elderly and patients are referred for physiotherapy weeks after the event, when they have become very immobile. The physiotherapist should always have a high index of suspicion of an underlying fracture if an elderly patient becomes increasingly immobile over a short period.

Fracture of the surgical neck of the humerus

Fracture of the surgical neck of the humerus results from a fall on the outstretched hand. The upthrust may shear off the greater tuberosity. Because the fragments are often impacted, a large tell-tale haematoma may be the first sign of the fracture. In the elderly, the shaft is usually impacted into the head of the humerus in an abducted position.

In the older person, because of impaction, reduction is unnecessary and unwise. Splinting is also unnecessary: the weight of the arm held in a sling tends to correct displacement. Union occurs in three weeks and consolidation in six weeks.

The soft-tissue injury is more important than the fracture because of the risk of development of a stiff shoulder. Even a marked deformity causes little interference with function. Early movement is the keynote to success (Wiles 1969). Pendular exercises of the shoulder must begin at once and the patient must be encouraged to abduct the arm actively as soon as possible. When giving passive treatment, the scapula should be fixed with one hand to ensure that true gleno-humeral movement is obtained.

Complications

1.*Stiff shoulder*. This is invariable if early movement has not been encouraged;

2.*Malunion*. This is not uncommon, but in the elderly causes little disability.

Patients may develop a reversed scapulo-humeral rhythm which may or may not interfere with function. It is a condition difficult to correct and correction will only succeed with considerable perseverance on the part of the patient and the physiotherapist. The aim is to commence treatment by giving the patient maximum sensory input to aid in correction and this is followed by a progressive reduction in input. Biofeedback may be of help. It is first essential to ensure that there is freedom of movement of the scapula.

In principle, re-education falls into six stages:

1. The patient is seated in front of a mirror, suitably dressed and the reversed pattern is shown; by comparison with the 'normal' side the patient must fully understand the deformity;
2. The patient is instructed to push the elbow down into the physiotherapist's hand which cups around the joint, in order to prevent elevation of the shoulder girdle. It is important NOT to place the hand over the patient's trapezius muscle as this will tend to make the patient elevate the shoulder girdle;
3. The patient is asked to abduct his arm, keeping the elbow pushed down into the physiotherapist's hand. The first sign of elevation of the shoulder girdle is pointed out to the patient and the arm is returned to the side and the procedure repeated;
4. The patient may attempt the same manoeuvre, but without vocal support and correction;
5. An attempt is made without vocal stimulus or the tactile stimulus from the physiotherapist's hand;
6. Finally, the patient attempts the correct pattern of movement without any stimulus.

EMG biofeedback from trapezius muscle can also be of value.

Colles' fracture

Colles' fracture results from a fall on the dorsiflexed hand, breaking the radius transversely just proximal to the wrist joint. The momentum of the body probably imposes a supinator force and the lower radius, with the hand, is twisted and tilted backwards and radially. The fracture is recognised by the classic 'dinner fork' deformity with prominence on the dorsum of the wrist and depression anteriorly.

Following reduction, the forearm is held in the pronated position, the wrist slightly palmarflexed and ulnar deviated and a plaster slab applied, which should extend from just below the elbow to the metacarpal necks and two-thirds of the way round the circumference of the wrist. The day following immobilisation, if the fingers are swollen, engorged or painful there should be no hesitation in splitting the bandage.

The fracture unites in six weeks and the slab may be discarded and replaced by a temporary crepe bandage. The patient should not be discharged from treatment following immobilisation before he can (a) comb his hair, (b) fully elevate the shoulder and (c) move his fingers freely. Regular active exercise of the shoulder, elbow and fingers must be insisted upon and a method of checking the procedure must be worked out with the patient or his relatives. Time spent on treatment during the period of immobilisation minimises the time required following removal of the plaster.

When the plaster is removed, return of the wrist and radio-ulnar movements is encouraged by active, functional and purposeful activity. It must be remembered that gripping power cannot be achieved unless there is an adequate range of extension at the wrist and rotation at the metacarpophalangeal joints; accessory movements are often required to ensure these movements are present.

Complications

1. *The circulation* in the fingers must be checked regularly.
2. *Stiffness* — shoulder stiffness may occur as a result of 'neglect' in the early stages following reduction. Similarly, finger stiffness is a sign of lack of adequate treatment.
3. *Sudeck's atrophy* — pain and stiffness of the finger joints appears a few weeks after injury. The fingers are puffy, patchily discoloured, unduly moist, hyperaesthetic and stiff. X-rays show patchy rarefaction of bones. With prolonged treatment for pain relief and with graduated exercises, recovery is slow but steady

over many months.

4. *Rupture* of the extensor pollicis longus tendon occasionally occurs a few weeks after an apparently trivial fracture. The patient should be aware and warned of this possibility and the physiotherapist should be alert to the signs which will present.

Falls and fracture of the femoral neck

Fracture of the femoral neck occurs mainly among older women. At any instant, about 50 per cent of acute orthopaedic beds are occupied by patients with fractured necks of femur (Grimley-Evans 1979). There is high morbidity and mortality associated with this injury.

The patient may fall, but often merely catches her foot while walking: the foot twists and the femoral neck is fractured by the rotation force. Osteoporosis and trabecular fatigue fractures may have weakened the bone and it may be the site of a secondary deposit. King (1986), in a study of 34 women and 10 men with fractured femoral necks attending hospitals in the Dublin area, discovered that most falls occurred during the day and during ordinary activities of domestic living. The highest incidence of falls occurred in the kitchen and very few falls occurred on the stairs. Locations of falls outside the home tended to be sited close to the house. The causes of falls are readily identified as slips, trips, loss of balance or 'drop attacks'. These can further be classified as accidental and non-accidental. Cape (1978) defined accidental falls as those that are precipitated by environmental factors and non-accidental falls as those that relate to the patient's condition.

It is very important that the physiotherapist should understand the relevance of falls in relation to fractures of the femoral neck in the elderly and should appreciate that such an understanding can help in the overall care and treatment of patients.

Sheldon (1960) and King (1986) have shown that most fractures of the neck of the femur caused by accidental falls occur as a result of slips and trips. Most of those who slip are aged between 65 and 74, whereas trips occur in those aged over 75. Brocklehurst (1978) and King (1986) report that there is a higher proportion of falls due to causes other than slipping in over-75 age group.

Extrinsic causes of falls have been identified as:

1. Wet floors;
2. Worn carpets;

3. Ice;
4. Inadequate lighting;
5. Broken footpaths;
6. Loose mats.

Footwear is often cited as a cause of falls. However, this is difficult to quantify, though it must be considered as an additional precipitating factor.

Distraction and lack of concentration such as might occur in a depressive condition or in a patient on psychotropic drugs can result in misinterpretation of environmental hazards, e.g. wet floors (Overstall 1980). Slow speed and a shorter step-length (Wild 1981), due to reduction in limb co-ordination with age and reduced move-ment of the pelvis, result in the foot being swung too low while walking and tripping may result.

Non-accidental falls are caused by loss of balance and 'drop attacks' and account for almost two-thirds of falls. Loss of balance may be initiated by extrinsic factors, e.g. a knock from another person or a dog, inadequate lighting and so on. However, intrinsic factors, related to the patient's condition may be the primary cause.

The centre of gravity of the human body lies in the region of the second sacral vertebra. If the body was a rigid object, then the vertical line through the centre of gravity should always fall within the support base if a fall is to be avoided. The body of course is not rigid, but made up of parts that are constantly moving and changing position on a very narrow support base. If the vertical line through the centre of gravity moves outside the support base, a whole range of compensatory mechanisms must be activated quickly if a fall is to be prevented. These mechanisms involve the use of visual, vestibular and proprioceptive information and an integrating centre in the brain, which sends corrective signals to appropriate muscles. During standing and walking, an individual's centre of gravity moves outside its support base. The corrective mechanism described above prevents the patient from falling. However, if these mechanisms are impaired as they may be in old age, the individual is more likely to fall (Isaacs 1982). An underlying illness will increase this tendency even further so that it is always very important to investigate a person who has a history of falls very thoroughly. There is a long list of possible aetiological factors which include poor vision, vertebrobasilar ischaemia, cervical spondy-losis, cardiac arrhythmias and postural hypotension. The cerebellum and brain stem have important roles in maintaining balance and it is not surprising that any interference with the blood supply may cause falls, for example, arteriosclerotic changes in the vertebrobasilar artery or external pressure on these arteries due to osteoarthritic changes in the cervical vertebrae will both produce similar problems. Falls or unsteadiness that occur on neck movement strongly suggest vertebrobasilar problems. 'Drop attacks' are thought to be due to vertebrobasilar ischaemia. The elderly person falls suddenly without warning and there is no loss of consciousness. He is then unable to stand without help. When assisted to stand, the neuronal pathways, which have been temporarily paralysed, are reactivated and the individual is able to get up. Sheldon (1960) described how pressure on the soles of the feet against a wall appeared to bring about a recovery of normal tone in anti-gravity muscles.

An ECG may reveal a cardiac abnormality and it is now possible to record a patient's ECG over a 24-hour period using a holter monitor. The monitor has an event marker, which the patient may activate if he/she feels unsteady. Subsequent analysis of the holter tape may reveal an occult cardiac arrythmia that can be treated.

The normal individual has corrective reflexes known as baro-reflexes to prevent fall of blood pressure on standing from a lying or seated position. Age changes in the autonomic nervous system often impair these reflexes. Many drugs such as tranquillisers, sedatives, hypotensive agents, diuretics and levodopa may cause a patient's blood pressure to drop on standing.

A fall due to postural hypotension usually occurs when the subject has walked a few feet from where he has been lying or sitting. Blood pressure should be measured in the lying position and again on standing and it is often useful to ask the patient to walk a few steps and then to measure the blood pressure again. A fall in systolic pressure greater than 20 mmHg (2.67 kPa) on standing is likely to be significant. Commonsense advice may be of great benefit to these patients. For instance, they should be told to get up gradually and to remain with their legs against the chair or bed for a short while before walking. A review of the medication may make a dramatic difference and elastic stockings may also help.

Physiotherapy and prevention of falls

Loss of balance is a cause of almost half of all falls. The role of the physiotherapist in the prevention of falls can be two-fold, 1. education and 2. treatment. Physiotherapists in either the hospital or the community setting have the necessary access to the elderly to carry out the roles of both educator and therapist.

Education. This may be divided into two areas: 1. explanation and 2. information. The cause of the fall should be explained so that a patient can understand what has happened or what might happen. Explanation can inspire confidence. The physiotherapist should inform the patient of the hazards associated with falls (the extrinsic factors). Patients should be encouraged to wear spectacles if prescribed and to attend the optician on a regular basis.

Prevention of extrinsic factors

1. Wet floors — wait until the floor has dried and is safe to walk on;
2. Lighting — have a lamp placed at the bedside or have a flashlamp at hand in case of emergency. Ensure that switches at the door are easily accessible;
3. Loose mats — remove or replace with non-slip mats;
4. Worn carpets — repair and remove all frayed ends;
5. Inadequate footwear — avoid wearing slippers around the house. Use proper shoes with gripped soles;
6. Stairs — should always be well-lit and carpeting, linoleum, checked for safety. Provision of handrail(s) is (are) essential;
7. Bathing — advice should be given about safety in bathing and appropriate aids should be supplied; co-operation with occupational therapists is important;
8. Outside — observe for hazards and advise on the avoidance of broken footpaths, ice; etc.

Assessment

Any patient who has been hospitalised with a fractured neck of femur due to a fall should be assessed for the cause of the fall. This information should provide an adequate basis for treatment and progression. For example, analysis of gait in a patient who had tripped might indicate the need for emphasis on exercises for hip-mobility and gait re-education. Assessment should include balance, posture, hip mobility and analysis of gait.

Exercise

The aims of exercise are:

1. To improve hip mobility bilaterally;

2. To improve postural control;
3. To re-educate gait, i.e. to increase the length of step and co-ordinate limb movement.

Hip mobility. Therapy should involve mobilising and strengthening exercises for both hips which would increase range of movement and strengthen specific muscles, e.g. the gluteus maximus. Exercises for particular muscle groups will be determined by the type of surgical intervention.

Postural control. Balance exercises should be incorporated into the standard physiotherapy treatment of all patients with a fractured femoral neck. Optimal stability may be achieved by a programme of exercises, progressing along the following lines:

1. Stability over a given base;
2. Ability to return to a stable position after disturbance;
3. Ability to move the trunk over a base;
4. Ability to move from one position to another;
5. Ability to balance over an unstable or moving base.

Analysis of Gait. On assessment, gait should be analysed for shortening and irregularity of step-length and the patient's ability to lift the feet adequately during the swing-through phase of walking. Patients should practise using stairs, especially those who will need to use stairs at home. Ideally, instruction on how to get up after falling should be given. Such treatment and explanation for 'fallers' should be incorporated into standard physiotherapy treatment of patients with fractured femoral necks. It should be remembered that many patients are often very confused and verbal instruction will have to be very clear.

Types of fractured femur

The fracture of the femoral neck may be subcapital, transcervical or basal (see Fig. 6.1). Garden (1971) has described four stages of displacement which may be correlated with prognosis:

Stage 1. Incomplete (abducted/impacted);
Stage 2. Complete without displacement.

Stages 1 and 2 give good results after internal fixation.

Figure 6.1: Fracture sites around the upper end of femur

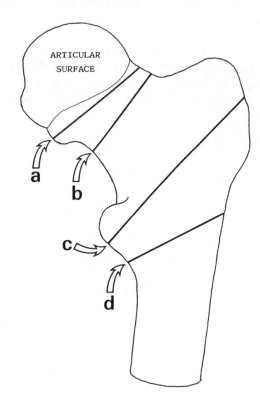

a. Subcapital
b. Transcervical
c. Intertrochanteric
d. Subtrochanteric

Stage 3. Complete with partial displacement;
Stage 4. Complete with full displacement.

Stages 3 and 4 have a high rate of non-union and avascular necrosis.
Fractures of the femoral neck have this poor capacity for healing because:

1. By tearing the capsular vessels, the injury deprives the head of the femur of its main blood supply;
2. Intra-articular bone has no contact with soft tissues, which

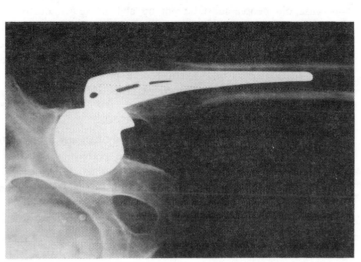

Figure 6.3: Austin–Moore prothesis used in a patient who had a subcapital fracture

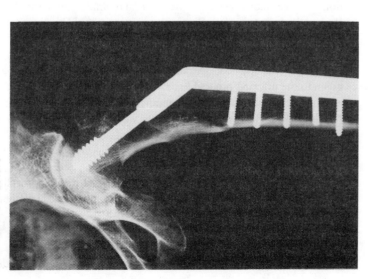

Figure 6.2: Dynamic hip screw used for fixation of a trochanteric fracture

could promote osteogenesis;

3. Synovial fluid prevents clotting of the fracture haematoma.

Apley (1976) considers that operative treatment is almost mandatory, because old people must be got up and active without delay if pulmonary complications and bed sores are to be avoided. Because of the morbidity associated with replacement, many surgeons favour internal fixation ('pin and plate' or dynamic hip screw) for trochanteric fractures (Fig. 6.2) and Austin-Moore prosthesis (Fig. 6.3) for subcapital and transcervical fractures in the elderly.

Treatment

In general, treatment is an emergency and often any pre-operative care is not possible. However, if time permits, instruction in breathing exercises is given, encouraging full respiratory movements.

Post-operatively, from the first day the patient should be encouraged to sit up in bed or in a chair, with the emphasis on activity. The patient should be encouraged to care for him/herself as much as possible and to follow through instructions that are given.

Breathing exercises and coughing will clear the lungs of secretions. Maintenance exercises for the uninjured leg are begun immediately, together with static quadriceps and gluteal activity on the injured leg. There is no evidence to show wasting or loss of power in the hamstring muscles, even after prolonged immobilisation. Active movements to the foot and ankle are carried out frequently during the day. Passive movements should be given to the patellae of both legs to avoid stiffness with consequent loss of mobility later.

From the second post-operative day, active/assisted exercises are given to the affected hip and knee. On about the tenth day, walking re-education is commenced, in conjunction with progressive balance re-education. The time for walking will vary from surgeon to surgeon and patient to patient. At no time following a pin and plate should the patient straight-leg raise with the injured leg as there is the danger of 'bending' the pin.

Stewart's (1965) classic monograph on the treatment approach to patients with fractured femoral necks still remains an excellent guide to the principles of care.

Complications

1. *General complications* — complications such as those that

follow any injury or operative procedures in the older person are liable to occur, especially deep-vein thrombosis, pulmonary embolism, pneumonia and bed sores.

2. *Avascular necrosis* — the blood supply to the head of the femur is disrupted and part or all of it dies.

3. *Non-union* — this is likely if the fracture line is unduly vertical, if the operation is performed with less than optimal skill, or if blood supply to the femoral head is diminished. Apley (1976) suggests that in the elderly, only two procedures should be considered: (a) if pain is not severe, a raised heel and stick or elbow crutch are sufficient; (b) if pain is considerable, total joint replacement may be performed.

Accidents in hospital

A survey of accidents in a geriatric department suggests that approximately 15 per cent of all elderly patients admitted to hospital will have an accident as an in-patient (Tinker 1979). In 40 per cent of accidents, ward furniture was implicated, particularly commodes, cotsides and geriatric chairs. Tinker advocated an urgent reappraisal of the design of all these items of furniture. She also emphasised the importance of reviewing equipment in a hospital on a regular basis. For instance, the brakes on beds, chairs and commodes are often ineffective. Frequently, rubber ferrules on chair legs are worn away, exposing the smooth metal, which has no grip on tiled flooring. Tinker has also emphasised the importance of proper footwear and clothing. Sloppy slippers and trailing dressing gowns are major hazards. Incorrect footwear can lead to immobility and can also be an accident hazard. Shoes should be carefully selected to suit the need of the individual. Most people will find that laced-up shoes with broad low heels are most suitable. Hospital chairs should vary in size to accommodate different patients with a range of disability and they should have arms to prevent sideways falls. An overzealous approach to encourage independence can itself lead to problems.

Good teamwork leading to active assessment of the patient's capabilities and disabilities should help reduce falls. It is interesting that relatively few falls occur in physiotherapy departments, even though patient activity is encouraged. Physiotherapists are trained to anticipate and therefore to prevent these problems. Although there are inherent risks in any rehabilitation programme, all reasonable steps must be taken to make the ward a safe environment for the patient (Coakley 1980).

REFERENCES

Aaron, J.E., Gallagher, J.C., Anderson, J., Stasink, L., Langton, B., Nordin, B.E.C. and Nicholson, M. (1974) 'Frequency of osteomalacia and osteoporosis in fractures of the proximal femur.' *Lancet, i* 229–33

Adler, S. (1985) 'Self care in the management of the degenerative knee joint.' *Physiotherapy,71*, 2, 58–60

Apley, A.G. (1982) *Apley's system of orthopaedics and fractures*, 6th edn, Butterworth Scientific, London

Badley, M., Lee, J. and Wood, P.H.N. (1979) 'Pattern of disability related to joint involvement in RA.' *Rheumatol. and Rehab., 18*, 105–9

Brewerton, D.A. (1979) 'Rheumatic disorders.' In I. Rossman (ed), *Clinical geriatrics*, Lippincott, Philadelphia

Brocklehurst, J.C. (1978) 'Fracture of the femur in old age.' *Age and ageing, 7*, 7–15

Caillet, R. (1971) *Hand pain and impairment*. F.A. Davis Co. Philadelphia

Cape, R. (1978) *Ageing: its complex management*. Harper and Row, New York

Chalmers, G.L. (1980) *Caring for the elderly sick*. Pitman Medical, Tunbridge Wells

Clarke, G.R., Willis, L.A., Stenner, L. and Nichols, P.J.R. (1974) 'Evaluation of physiotherapy in the treatment of osteoarthrosis of the knee.' *Rhematol. and Rehab. 13*, 190–7

Coakley, D. (1980) 'On the dangers of getting out of bed in hospital.' *Health trends, 12*, 5–6

Cuddigan, J.H.P. and Mathews, J.A. (1971) 'The shoulder–hand syndrome.' *Physiotherapy, 57*, 1, 25–7

Ekblom, B., Lovgren, O., Alderin, M., Fridstrom, M. and Satterstrom, G. (1975) 'Effect of short-term training on patients with rheumatoid arthritis.' *Scan. J. Rheumatol., 4*, 80–5

Exton-Smith, A.N. (1983) 'Integration of geriatric and general medical services.' *J. Am. Geriat. Soc, 12*, 810–11

Exton-Smith, A.N. and Overstall, P. (1979) *Geriatrics*. MTP Press, Lancaster

Garden, R.S. (1971) 'Malreduction and avascular necrosis in sub-capital fractures of the femur.' *J. Bone and Jt. Surg. 53 B*, 183–97

Goffman, E. (1968) *Stigma: notes on the management of spoiled identity*. Penguin Books, Harmondsworth

Grimley-Evans, J. (1979) 'Fractured proximal femur in Newcastle-upon-Tyne.' *Age and Ageing, 8*, 16–24

Helal, B. (1965) 'The pain in primary osteoarthrosis of the knee.' *Postgrad. Med. J., 41*, 172–81

Hodkinson, H.M. (1971) 'Scleroderma in the elderly with special reference to the CRST syndrome.' *J.Am.Ger. Soc., 19*, 224–8

Hyde, S.A. (1980) *Physiotherapy in rheumatology* Blackwell Scientific Publications, Oxford

Isaacs, B. (1982) 'Disorders of balance.' In F.I. Caird, (ed), *Neurological disorders in the elderly*, Wright, Bristol

Jahss, M.H. (1979) 'Geriatric aspects of the foot and ankle.' In I. Rossman (ed), *Clinical Geriatrics*, Lippincott, Philadelphia

Kessel, L. and Watson, M. (1977) 'The Painful Arc Syndrome.' *J. Bone and Jt. Surge. 59B*, 166–72

King, S. (1986) 'The extrinsic causes of falls resulting in fractured neck of femur', Project submitted, School of Physiotherapy, University of Dublin

Maitland, G.D. (1977) *Peripheral manipulation*. Butterworth Scientific, London

Meenan, R.F., Yelin, E.H. and Nevitt, M. (1981) 'Impact of chronic disease.' *Arthritis and Rheum. 24*, 544–9

Nordemar, R., Berg, U., Ekblom, B. and Edstrom, L. (1976) 'Changes in muscle fibre size and physical performance in patients with rheumatoid arthritis after 7 months physical training.' *Scand. J. Rheumat., 5*, 233–7

Overstall, P.W. (1980) 'Prevention of falls in the elderly.' *J. Am. Ger. Soc. 28*, 481–3

Partridge, R.E.H. and Duthie, J.J.R. (1963) 'Controlled trials of the effect of complete immobilisation of the joints in rheumatoid arthritis.' *Ann. of Rheum. Dis., 22*, 91–9

Sheldon, J.H. (1960) 'On the natural history of falls in old age.' *Brit. Med. J., 2*, 1685–90

Slannka, J. (1980) 'Difficult Disease — Difficult Patient.' *J. Gerontol. Nursing, 6*, 94

Steinbrocher, O. and Argyros, T.D. (1958) 'The shoulder–hand syndrome: present status as a diagnostic and therapeutic entity.' *The Med. Clinics of N. America, 42*, 1533

Steward, M.A. (1965) *Rehabilitation following fractures of the femoral neck*. Heinemann, London

Tinker, G.M. (1979) 'Accidents in a geriatric department.' *Age and Ageing, 8*, 196–8

Wadsworth, H. and Chanmugam, A.P. (1983) *Electrophysical agents in physiotherapy*, 2nd edn, Science Press, New South Wales

Wagstaff, P.S., Wagstaff S.J. and Downey, M. (1986) 'A pilot study to compare the efficacy of continuous and pulsed magnetic energy (short wave diathermy) in the relief of low back pain.' *Physiotherapy, 72*, 11, 563–6

Wild, D. (1981) 'How dangerous are falls in old people at home?' *Brit. Med. J., 2*, 266–8

Wiles, P. (1969) *Fractures dislocations and sprains*, 2nd edn, J. and A. Churchill Ltd, London

Wright, V. and Owen, S. (1976) 'The effect of rheumatoid arthritis on the social situation of housewives.' *Rheumat. and Rehab., 15*, 156–60

7

Cardiac and Peripheral Vascular Rehabilitation

Cardiac enlargement is common in older people, indeed the left ventricular wall may be some 25 per cent thicker at the age of 80 than at the age of 30 (Sjogren 1971). The heart valves become stiffer with age (McMillan and Lev 1964). There is no doubt that with a maximal load, both heart rate and stroke volume are decreased, with a resultant reduction in cardiac output (Brandfonbrener, Landowne and Shock 1955) and the time required for the heart rate to return to normal is prolonged (Montoye, Willis and Cunningham 1968).

Ageing arteries show progressive chemical and anatomical changes that are directly related to alteration in function. The elastin content diminishes with ageing and the collagen content increases. With increasing vascular rigidity, the systolic blood pressure rises; the diastolic pressure also increases.

The normal ageing heart is well able to provide adequate output because requirement is reduced. However, there is progressive loss of ability to deal with stress. Sudden increase in heart rate, anoxia and decreased venous return may cause congestive cardiac failure, coronary insufficiency or myocardial necrosis.

SYMPTOMS AND SIGNS OF CARDIAC DISEASE IN THE ELDERLY

Dyspnoea on effort is one of the most common features of cardiac disease in the elderly. If there is marked cardiac failure, the patient may be breathless lying down (orthopnoea) and may become acutely dyspnoeic during the night (paroxysmal nocturnal dyspnoea). In many elderly patients, respiratory and cardiac disease co-exist.

Ankle oedema is a feature of cardiac failure, but it is very important to remember that there are many other causes of oedema in the elderly. Other evidence must be present before attributing oedema to cardiac failure. Stasis oedema is probably the most common cause of ankle swelling in the older patient. It may first be seen some days after the patient has been admitted to hospital. Many elderly patients are terrified in the environs of a busy hospital ward so they stay seated by their bed. Diuretic therapy in this situation is quite inappropriate and it may lead to postural hypotension. The correct procedure is to mobilise the patient. There are other causes of ankle oedema such as anaemia, fluid-retaining drugs like phenylbutazone, venous obstruction, cellulitis and malnutrition.

Cyanosis is another sign of a low cardiac output in the elderly. The tissues extract the available oxygen from the haemoglobin and the resulting reduced haemoglobin gives a bluish tinge to the tissues. The patient may have blue lips, cheeks and extremities. Cyanosis can also be seen in patients with severe respiratory disease. In patients with peripheral vascular disease, cyanosis may be observed in the extremities.

Chest pain is an unusual cardiac sign in old age. Myocardial infarction does not often present with the crushing central chest pain radiating to the neck and left arm seen commonly in younger patients. It may present as chest discomfort, dyspnoea, fatigue, acute confusion, a stroke or sudden loss of consciousness.

Faints and falls may be caused by cardiac problems. They may be due to postural hypotension, arrythmias or myocardial infarction. The patient with arrythmias may also complain of palpitations. The heart may be beating too quickly (tachycardia) or too slowly (bradycardia) to maintain an adequate cardiac output.

MYOCARDIAL INFARCTION

The risk factors for coronary artery disease are altered in the elderly. Obesity of a major degree is unusual in those of advanced years. Total cholesterol is no longer a risk factor in men over 65 (Gordon *et al.* 1977). The type A personality described by Rosenham (1970) — hard-driving, competitive, time-conscious, loses statistical significance as a risk factor in the elderly. Smoking is to be discouraged whatever the age of the individual.

The mortality of acute myocardial infarction is not easily determined in the elderly; however, it is true that there is an approximately equal sex distribution (Biorck 1968). In younger groups those who survive the first day of hospitalisation have a three-to-one chance of survival; in the aged, the chance of survival is less than one in four (Thould 1965). Williams *et al*. (1976) showed that those who are admitted to a coronary care unit do better. Although absolute survival after infarctions is shorter in older than in younger groups, if comparisons of remaining life expectancy are made between survivors of a myocardial infarct and the uninvolved population of the same age, the mortality risk is greater in younger persons. In other words, life expectancy is less adversely affected in the older person (Biorck 1968).

Treatment

The treatment of acute myocardial infarction in the elderly is similar to that for younger ages. Hadi, Morris and Kicher (1980) advocate early ambulation and reassurance, with discharge some seven to ten days after admission. A typical regime is as follows:

All cases from admission and until mobile have leg, arm and breathing exercises, initially aimed at the prevention of deep-vein thrombosis, the maintenance of mobility and good air entry. Day 1 is taken as the day on which pain ceases.

Day 1. Sit out for 30 minutes;

Day 2. Sit out for 30–60 minutes, morning and afternoon; a few steps with supervision; commence ward exercises;

Day 3. Sit out for one hour, morning and afternoon; walk to bathroom with supervision; ward exercises continue;

Day 4. Sit out for two hours morning and afternoon; increase walking distance;

Day 5. Out for most of the time; take a few steps on the stairs;

Day 6. Walk at a leisurely pace as required; attempt one flight of stairs supervised;

Day 7. Extend walking distance; attempt one flight of stairs at a slightly quicker pace;

Days 8 to 10. Discharge?

Ward exercises

Standing at the bed end:

1. Hold bed end — double knee-bends;

2. Arms by side — raise arms to shoulder level and lower;
3. Hold bed end — alternate leg-swinging;
4. Arms by side — arm-circling.

Repeat the exercises three to four times on day 2, progressing to eight to ten repetitions over the next days.

Patients should be informed that increased anxiety after leaving hospital is common. Weakness, faintness, undue breathlessness and chest pain during exercise are indications to rest and, if persistent, should be reported to the patient's doctor.

Rehabilitation following discharge

First week at home.

1. Ten hours in bed at night;
2. One to two hours rest after lunch;
3. If able, climb the stairs once daily;
4. Stay mobile indoors and do not encourage visitors.

Second week.

1. Rest as before;
2. Climb the stairs three to four times a day;
3. Walk out of doors.

Third week. If possible, increase the length of walking outdoors at a gentle pace for one or two miles.

COR PULMONALE

Acute cor pulmonale with right-heart failure is usually precipitated by pulmonary infarction due to pulmonary embolus. Chronic cor pulmonale develops commonly as a result of chronic bronchitis and emphysema. The typical patient is a male with a long history of smoking, repeated respiratory infections, cough, shortness of breath on effort and attacks of wheezing. When right-heart failure develops, the neck veins become distended and peripheral oedema is evident. Treatment is on the lines appropriate to a younger person. From a physiotherapist's point of view, breathing exercises are given to encourage maximal expansion, especially diaphragmatic, lateral-costal and posterior-basal expansion. Postural drainage may be required.

HYPERTENSION

Mean systolic and diastolic pressures rise with age so that it is not uncommon to see a diastolic pressure of 100 mmHg (13.3 kPa) and a systolic pressure of 180 mmHg (24 kPa). There is considerable debate in the medical literature as to the correct management of hypertension in elderly patients. Most agree that very severe hypertension should be treated, but there is less agreement in the case of mild and moderate hypertension. Treatment is not without side effects and falls due to postural hypotension are not uncommon in elderly patients taking anti-hypertensive agents.

VENOUS THROMBOSIS

Venous thrombosis and pulmonary embolism are being encountered with increasing frequency in the elderly. The reasons for this increasing incidence are the longer survival of critically ill patients and more extensive surgical procedures carried out in the elderly.

Venous thrombosis may involve the superficial or deep veins. Superficial-vein thrombosis is seen often in patients with varicose veins who are immobilised. There is local redness and tenderness and the thrombosed veins may be palpable. The patients need not be immobilised and the condition usually settles with bandaging and anti-inflammatory agents. If the patient has to be immobilised for some other reason, he should be given isometric exercises to encourage the circulation.

Deep-vein thrombosis is a serious complication of many illnesses that immobilise elderly patients. Coon (1977) identified the following risk factors for deep-vein thrombosis:

1. Past history;
2. Immobilisation for longer than one week;
3. Obesity;
4. Hemiplegia or other causes of enforced immobility;
5. Heart disease;
6. Carcinoma of lung, gastrointestinal tract and genitourinary tract;

7. Major surgery (fractures, abdominal).

Deep-vein thrombosis is serious because of the risk of embolus formation leading to a life-threatening pulmonary infarction. The patient may complain of calf pain and there is usually warmth and swelling of the affected limb. Ankle oedema may also be present and dorsiflexion of the foot may produce calf pain (Homan's sign). Physiotherapists, if they are vigilant, may diagnose deep-vein thrombosis in the early stages. The diagnosis may be confirmed by Doppler or radioisotope scanning of the limb.

Treatment

Initial treatment is with anticoagulation and elevation of the bed will be required. Elevation of the extremity is essential in order to provide venous drainage. The correct procedure is elevation and head down. If a patient is treated at home, the foot end of the bed needs to be raised by 30 to 40 cm; use of pillows alone might interfere with venous drainage. If the head-up position is necessary, great care must be taken to ensure that there is not over flexion at the hip which may cause inadequate drainage of the iliac vessels; this could cause iliac stasis and possible iliac thrombosis.

Avoidance of deep-breathing and straining should be stressed in the acute stage, especially if emboli are suspected. After the acute phase, active dorsiflexion and plantarflexion are given, and early mobilisation is encouraged.

It will often be found that elderly patients are given low-dose anticoagulant drugs as a preventive measure, especially if undergoing surgical procedures. Patients should be given exercise pre-operatively and, of course, early post-operative mobilisation is essential.

VENOUS LEG ULCER

Once ulceration has occurred in the lower limbs, it requires costly, time-consuming effort to put it right, yet many ulcers could be prevented (Parbhoo 1979).

The lower extremity is a common site for pruritic dermatitis. Swelling of the legs from any cause, congestive failure or incompetence of the venous system with varicose veins, impairs diffusion of nutrients to the skin. This causes a mild eczematous reaction, aggravated by scratching. Scratching causes a break in the skin, with superficial infection. The patient should be informed and told not to scratch. Emphasis should be placed on simple hygiene and nail care.

Patients require education about footwear. Claw toes and depressed metatarsal heads are deformities frequently found in the avascular foot. As mentioned in Chapter 6, metatarsal pads need to be individually made and fitted. The risk is that an ill-fitting pad will push the proximal interphalangeal joint against the shoe. Calluses form and then an ulcer.

A re-education programme should stress the importance of a daily foot inspection for cuts, bruises and skin breakdown and the need to wash and dry the feet carefully. The elderly should avoid extremes of temperature in all bathing and should be warned of the dangers of warming cold feet and legs by electric fires. Socks, tights and stockings must fit properly and garters should not be worn. Chemical gels to remove corns should be avoided. New shoes need to be broken in gradually. Advice should be given on how to cut nails. Therapists have long been accustomed to antenatal classes, kinetic-handling classes for back care, sports-training, etc., — all groups aimed at the prevention of injury. There should be similar prevention classes for the elderly.

In the elderly, ulcers are slow to heal, often requiring prolonged care. The objectives of physiotherapy care are:

1. To relieve pain;
2. To control infection;
3. To promote healing;
4. To reduce oedema;
5. To improve circulation;
6. To mobilise all parts of the limb and ulcer.

Pain is often present and it may be due to oedema in the limb. It is important that during treatment to the limb other than to the ulcer area, the ulcer itself is protected, for example by a Eusol pack. The oedema is relieved by elevation of the limb for about 20 minutes prior to active treatment. Interferential therapy (1–100 Hz and 1–10 Hz), in conjunction with intermittent compression, is a useful method of relieving oedema. In various centres in France, particularly at the Corentin Celton Hospital in Paris under Professor Garbay, promising results at reduction of oedema and wound-healing are being recorded using Therafield (640 Hz for one hour). Pulsed short-wave diathermy may be used.

Mobility of skin and connective tissue is regained by connective-tissue rolling. The thickened areas are easily palpable. Finger-kneading must be given to the coulisses (hollows behind the malleoli). Effleurage, deeply and slowly to the whole limb (commencing proximally), completes massage (Bannister 1968). Foot and ankle dorsiflexion and plantarflexion and quadriceps contractions aid both mobility in the limb and venous return. If infection is absent, ultrasound may be used to relieve oedema and break down adhesions. Low dosage for a short period is known to promote healing. Doses of up to 1.5 Wcm^{-2} for three to four minutes active-treatment time are advocated.

Whichever treatment is chosen for the ulcer, a tracing should be taken at each treatment; this provides an accurate assessment of progress. The ulcer is cleaned with Eusol and dried. A double piece of 'cellophane' larger than the ulcer is sterilised by wiping it thoroughly with ether on both sides. This is placed on the ulcer and the margin is traced using a fine-point felt pen. The 'cellophane' is removed and the lower layer, which has been in contact with the ulcer, is discarded and the tracing kept as a record. The orientation must be marked upon the tracing as ulcers may change shape (Savage 1960), see Fig. 7.1. The area may be calculated using graph paper.

Figure 7.1: Tracing of a venous leg ulcer

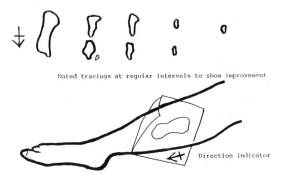

Dated tracings at regular intervals to show improvement

Direction indicator

TRACING OF A VENOUS LEG ULCER

The ulcer itself may be treated by ultraviolet irradiation. If the ulcer is indolent, a strong reaction is required to destroy devitalised cells. An E_4 is given to the base of the ulcer. Care must be taken, by masking, to avoid irradiation of new epithelial and granulation tissue. The surrounding area of skin is irradiated with an E_1 to improve circulation. Some good initial results have been obtained using IR laser. The laser head is moved around the margin of each ulcer area for three minutes and treatment given daily.

Wearing a sterile glove, the region of the ulcer may be treated with deep frictions to soften the induration, working inwards towards the edges of the ulcer itself. The ulcer may be moved from side-to-side with modified wringing.

Local medications are varied and will depend upon the physician in charge. The object of the local medication is to create sterile conditions in which optimum cellular activity and wound contraction may take place. Barton and Barton (1981) recommend Disadine or Cetavlex cream.

On completion of care of the ulcer, a compression bandage must be applied in order to maintain and gain still further reduction in oedema. A sorbo pad or Plastazote pad is applied over the dressing, of a size corresponding to the ulcer and the oedematous area around it. Padding is placed in the coullises and round the lower leg and foot. Over this, a bandage of elastic webbing (3–4 m) is applied in the Bisgaard method, see fig 7.2. It starts from under the medial side of the sole, is carried once straight around the foot, then upwards and outwards over the dorsum, around the back of the heel just above the calcaneal tubercle, outwards and downwards across the dorsum and under the sole, near the heel. The bandage must extend to the popliteal fossa as a simple spiral. The patient or relatives should be shown how to bandage. However, this is often a confusing procedure for the patient.

The patient's gait is re-educated and he should be given simple home exercises for foot and ankle to maintain mobility and to encourage venous return.

PERIPHERAL ARTERIAL DISEASE

The peripheral circulation of certain older patients is impaired because of gradual narrowing of the arteries due to atherosclerosis. Atherosclerosis is caused by deposition of lipid material in the vessel walls. Diabetes and cigarette-smoking are factors that predispose to

Figure 7.2: The Bisgaard technique

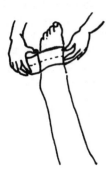 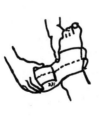 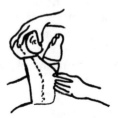

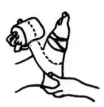 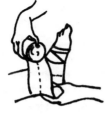 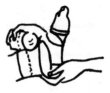

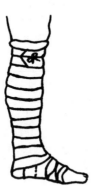

Source: Wale 1961

the condition.

Initially, the patient may notice calf pain on walking (intermittent claudication) and coldness of the legs. With progression of the disease, the patient may complain of pain (especially in the foot) when at rest. It is particularly severe at night and the patient may experience relief by hanging his foot out of the bed. The feet may appear discoloured. Gangrene may develop if there is further deterioration in the circulation.

Treatment

Local infection will increase the demands on the circulation and may precipitate gangrene. It is therefore very important that foot hygiene should be very good. Diabetics should always be advised about the importance of good foot care. Any infection should be treated promptly with antibiotics. Patients who smoke should be advised to stop although, surprisingly, this advice is often ignored. The patients should be seen by a vascular surgeon at an early stage if possible, as a lumbar sympathectomy or vascular reconstruction may be indicated. Non-weight-bearing exercises for the limbs may improve circulation and in less-advanced cases, intermittent positive pressure leggings may be used in an effort to reduce oedema and encourage limb drainage. Adequate relief of pain with analgesics is an important aspect of management.

Because of the progressive nature of the condition, many of the patients come ultimately to amputation.

Amputation

The level of amputation is decided by the surgeon. Robinson (1976) found that with above-knee amputations, hospital mortality was in the area of 30 per cent and only 18 per cent of patients were discharged walking adequately, whereas with below-knee amputations there was a 14 per cent mortality and 73 per cent of patients were discharged walking adequately. A better understanding of the peripheral vascular problems and the more intensive use of reconstruction arterial procedures has favoured the choice of lower levels. The decision as to which level can only be made after careful study of each patient. Factors influencing the decision are the extent of gangrene and ulceration, the degree of infection, the condition of adjacent areas, the degree of arterial impairment and the severity of the pain.

The treatment plan may vary considerably with each individual. Rehabilitation begins at the pre-operative stage, as development of rapport between the physiotherapist and the patient is essential. The patient will require reassurance that the operation will rid him of pain, which is often the immediate concern and leave him with minimal loss of function, which is the long-term aim. Unless these two facts can be reconciled, the post-operative care is going to be difficult. Studies on survival after amputation have not been very encouraging and a realistic picture must be presented to relatives. Approximately 45 per cent of elderly amputees will not survive more than one year and only a few will survive for five years. As many as 30 per cent of those who do survive will require amputation of the other leg.

The primary aim for the elderly is to achieve safe function in the activities of daily living (Engstrom and Van de Ven 1985). A few relevant exercises are repeated in the same way every day. Treatment sessions are kept short and must include balance and transfer activities; stump exercises are of secondary importance.

Several years ago, it was considered that the majority of elderly amputees would discard their prostheses soon after discharge from hospital. However, Katrak and Baggot (1980) consider this untrue and showed that 79 per cent of their patients were successful prosthesis users and that rehabilitation and mobility were maintained at home. These results concur with those of Steinberg, Garcia and Rositger (1974) and Clarke and Blue (1983) who demonstrated optimistic results among elderly amputees following rehabilitation.

Pre-operative procedures

Before the operation, the physiotherapist should see both the patient and his family to answer questions about post-operative care (Burgess and Alexander 1973). Mensch and Ellis (1982) suggest that pre-operative assessment should include examination of the patient's:

1. Respiratory condition;
2. Arm strength;
3. Remaining leg strength;
4. Sensation in the lower extremities;
5. Trunk strength;
6. Ability to transfer.

127

Activities to improve strength in preparation for post-operative care is important. Discretion should be used, as toxicity, due to gangrenous changes, or the patient's state, or pain, may hinder a full programme.

A light-weight frame should be measured for the patient and labelled with his name prior to surgery. The patient is shown how to transfer from bed to chair or commode. Active exercises are given to the normal leg. Quadriceps and gluteal contractions and adductor activity are practised in preparation for post-operative care. These are positive approaches towards reassurance.

Post-operative activity

Immediately after the operation, the general condition of the patient should be ascertained from the ward sister or doctor.

1. Respiratory care. Every effort must be made to avoid static pneumonia.

2. Trunk exercises. In the elderly, a modified exercise regime is necessary. It should attempt to balance abdominal and back extensor activity so as to improve posture and thus balance when sitting and standing.

3. Exercises for the normal leg. The remaining limb is going to be the dominant limb in walking activity and so full-range mobility and strengthening is of great importance. Early activity in bed will both assist nurses and help to prevent the formation of deep-vein thrombosis as well as pneumonia.

4. Balance activity. The patient is taught how to move himself about in bed. Balance when sitting is gained first; this gives the patient confidence for the later attempt to stand. Unless balance in the seated position can be achieved, it is unwise to attempt to stand the patient.

When the patient stands for the first time, he should be warned of the possibility of a 'throbbing' sensation or 'feeling his leg fill with blood' in the amputated limb and he should be advised that this is quite normal and will slowly wear off. At first, standing balance is achieved in a walking frame. The length of treatment initially will be guided by (a) the patient's tolerance and (b) the surgeon.

5. The stump.

(a) Exercises. Muscle contractions of the hip extensors prepare the patient for standing. In the above-knee amputee, they help reduce the risk of flexion-contracture and in a below-knee amputee, hip-extension will ultimately be necessary to lock the artificial knee into extension. It is essential that the patient realises that the hip extensors are working and not any other compensatory groups of muscles.

Quadriceps contraction in a below-knee amputee should be begun at once. Again, it is essential to ensure that it is the quadriceps muscles that are active and not other muscles.

In the above-knee amputee, emphasis is placed on hip-adductor activity to counteract the likely deformity. However, it should be remembered that hip-abductor activity is of importance because of the influence of this muscle group on the pelvis and thus on gait.

The later post-operative care of the stump and patient is very variable in different centres. Rigid dressings, non-removable casts, fabricated socks, etc., are all advocated. Alexander (1975) does not favour the practice of initiating ambulation immediately following surgery, because of the risk of stump breakdown or splitting the suture line.

(b) Observation. The physiotherapist should examine the stump for pressure areas, colour of skin, temperature of skin, patellar mobility (in below-knee amputees), range of movement and oedema.

It should be remembered that not all elderly patients will be suitable for a prosthesis (McCollough 1971). Pre-existing neurological or other medical problems, the presence of a previous amputation, or the failure of tissue to heal may make the fitting of a prosthesis unrealistic. A wheelchair should be provided in these cases. It should be remembered that certain elderly patients, especially those who are frail, may manage better at home in a wheelchair and also maintain a good 'quality of life'.

Gait re-education

It is essential that all patients attend a physiotherapy department for gait re-education immediately following delivery of the temporary prosthesis. If there is delay, there is a risk that an amputee may attempt to use the prosthesis and as a result produce a poor walking pattern. The elderly patient is likely to sit and wait for something to happen so that delay will result in a deterioration of their physical and mental condition. The physiotherapist must keep in touch with the patient whether he is at home or in hospital.

Plans for transport to the physiotherapy department must be

made. If, because of transport difficulties, a patient cannot attend for gait re-education, then arrangements must be made for such treatment to take place at another centre. Such arrangements are not always easy, but it is essential that perseverance is maintained until suitable appointments are made.

Regardless of age, daily treatment is preferred. This should take place during a whole morning or afternoon so that suitable rest periods my be permitted. The advantages of daily care outweigh the disadvantages associated with travel. Continuity of care improves the prosthetic re-education and the daily wearing of the 'limb' helps the patient to accept the 'device'. Skin over the stump tends to toughen more quickly. Activities of daily living which encourage the patient should be carried out. The aim for the elderly amputee is to attain the best possible gait pattern, whilst appreciating that certain physical problems such as contractures impose limitations.

It is important to check that the patient can put on and take off his prosthesis correctly and that the clothing worn is suitable. Walking commences between parallel bars with the patient dressed in outdoor clothes. After initial instruction, the patient may be left to practise on his own, but making sure that adequate rest periods are taken. Mirrors can be a helpful adjunct to treatment as they give visual feedback on progress. When a patient can manage safely in parallel bars, progression is made to a frame, or ideally, walking sticks. It is important that walking does not become an end in itself, but that walking is linked to activities of daily living. Following discharge, further assessment or treatment is usually only required if a new prosthesis is ordered.

Many elderly amputees have multiple medical problems; treatment aims at safety and function. A home assessment is essential so that treatment will be relevant to the patient's needs. The patient must not only learn to walk safely, but must be able to stand from the seated position and vice versa. A fall is a catastrophe for the elderly amputee. The selection of the appropriate walking aid is important; for many patients, the frame will remain the aid of choice. Once a prosthesis is fitted comfortably and the patient is safe when walking, the community physiotherapist should be contacted so that activity in the home can commence.

The bilateral amputee

In common with younger patients with bilateral amputation, elderly patients, if they walk will do so with a wide base. The patient is taught how to put on and take off the artificial limbs. This requires time, patience, perseverance and much practice. The patient then dresses and commences walking between parallel bars. Standing and sitting can be very difficult and it is important to experiment in order to find the most suitable type of chair. The energy required to use two prostheses is very high and time must be allowed for patients to have frequent rest periods. Bilateral amputees should not be allowed to walk with a frame as the base is rarely wide enough and the patient tends to fall backwards while lifting the frame. The choice for the older patient will nearly always be quadrupods. For the older patient, a wheelchair may be recommended at an early stage.

Dressing

Most elderly patients need help or guidance, particularly with trousers and underpants. The hemiplegic or bilateral, lower-limb amputee may need special aids or adaptations for dressing. It is important to note that if it is still impossible for a patient to put on underpants or trousers independently after daily dressing-practice, it is very unlikely that the independent application of a prosthesis will be possible.

Wheelchairs

After a method of transfer has been established, the patient must be taught to manoeuvre the chair safely. The brakes and footrests must be explained, demonstrated and fully understood by the patient and any helper. The axis of the rear wheels needs to be set back to compensate for loss of body weight in the front; anti-tipping devices will replace the patient's foot. Sitting boards need to be fitted for both above- and below-knee amputees. The above-knee amputee must avoid pelvic drop and the below-knee amputee rests with the knee in extension. A stump board must be provided for through-knee and below-knee stumps; this will protect the stump from knocks, prevent contracture of the knee joint and control oedema. Patients with poor eyesight, hearing, weak hands or arms and poor sensation, require lengthy instruction and practice. The confused patient will need constant supervision.

Stump oedema

Stump oedema occurs immediately after the operation as a result of surgical trauma and may also recur at any time. It is important that the physiotherapist recognises the total problem so that the patient may appreciate the difficulty and learn how to cope.

1. *Elevation.* The foot of the bed may be elevated, providing blood pressure is stable and the vascularity of the other limb and stump are adequate.

2. *Exercise.* Active contraction of the stump muscles is the best method of reducing oedema. The below-knee amputee must imagine the performance of alternate dorsiflexion and plantarflexion, and the through- and above-knee amputee must perform alternate hip flexion and extension and hip abduction and adduction. These active exercises must be performed at regular intervals throughout the day.

3. *Bandaging.* Very few elderly patients will be able to apply a bandage themselves. There are probably more risks associated with poor bandaging than there are benefits.

4. *Intermittent variable air-pressure machines.* There are a variety of machines available, but the general principle is that by varying air pressure around the stump in a pre-determined cyclic fashion, the circulation of blood and lymph can be modified with beneficial results.

5. *Shrinker socks.* These elasticated stump socks are available in a variety of sizes from limb-fitting centres. They are less likely to wrinkle and cause a tourniquet effect than other elasticated materials, as the exact size may be made available. When worn first, the sock should be tried for half an hour under supervision. The stump is observed during this time for colour change and indentation, which may indicate that the sock is not the right size. The sock should only be worn when the patient is awake but not wearing the prosthesis.

Stump care

Alexander (1979) suggests;

1. The stump should be washed daily and with warm water to avoid a build-up of salt deposits;
2. The stump must be dried carefully to leave the skin smooth;
3. Skin folds should be cleansed with cotton wool swabs to eliminate bacterial growth;
4. Any abrasions should be reported;
5. If possible, the patient is taught to examine the stump with a mirror, but many elderly patients will rely upon a relative, helper or nurse. Below-knee amputees should note the tibial tubercle and fibular head; above-knee amputees should look at the skin both in the groin area and near the distal end of the femur.

Pain relief

Transcutaneous electrical nerve stimulation (TENS) may be of some assistance in reducing or controlling chronic pain in the stump and also phantom pain. The mechanism of working is possibly by the pain-gate theory or through the release of endorphins during stimulation. Interferential therapy (90–100 Hz or 100–32 Hz) treatment can bring considerable relief of pain and diadynamic (ultra-reiz) treatment may be used. O'Connell (1984) found that the effects of interferential would last up to 2 months, though at least 7 treatments were required before relief was initially obtained. A vibrator has been shown to give a patient temporary relief of pain. Ultrasound has been used in an attempt to reduce pain due to neuromas, but with questionable results. If, during healing, scar tissue becomes adherent to the underlying tissue, mobilisation of these tissues may be brought about by frictions. Frictions are not carried out over oedematous skin areas or if inflammation is present.

Housing

The elderly patient may well have an immediate housing problem that will require early and active assessment. Any delay may result in prolonged hospitalisation for the patient and deterioration in the patient's overall state. A home visit with the medical social worker and occupational therapist should take place and if necessary, the local authority should be contacted. Under the Chronically Sick and Disabled Persons Act 1970, local authorities are obliged to seek suitable housing for the disabled person.

Sport and leisure activity

The physiotherapist can advise about sport and leisure activities, but advice must be realistic with regard to age and condition. The main considerations before starting an activity are that the stump should be well-healed and toughened, that the general muscle strength should be reasonable and that stamina is adequate.

Darts may be enjoyed either in the seated or standing position. Bowls may be played outdoors or indoors from a wheelchair or when using a prosthesis. Fishing can be enjoyed from the wheelchair as well as in a sitting or standing position. However, it is unlikely that one will make a sportsman out of an individual who has always led a sedentary life. What is important is to show the amputee that there are many activities that may still be pursued despite amputation.

133

REFERENCES

Alexander, A. (1975) *Amputees guide, below the knee*. Medic. Publ. Co., New York

────── (1979) 'The dysvascular amputee. Surgery and rehabilitation.' *Curr. Prob. Surg.* 1

Bannister, C.R. (1968) 'Physiotherapy in the treatment of venous leg ulcers.' *Physiotherapy, 54*, 8, 272-5

Barton, A and Barton, M (1981) *Prevention in the management and prevention of pressure sores*. Faber and Faber, London

Biorck, G. (1968) 'The biology of myocardial infarction.' *Circulation, 37*, 1071-973

Brandfonbrener, M., Landowne, M and Shock, N.W. (1955) 'Changes in cardiac output with age.' *Circulation, 12*, 577

Burgess, F.M. and Alexander, A. (1973) 'The expanding role of the physical therapist in the amputee rehabilitation team.' *Phys. Ther. 53*, 141-4

Clarke, G.S. and Blue, B. (1983) 'Rehabilitation of elderly amputees.' *J. Am. Ger. Assoc., 31,7*, 439-48

Coon, W.N. (1977) 'Epidemiology of venous thromboembolism.' *Ann. Surg. 186*, 149-52

Engstrom, B. and Van de Ven, C. (1985) *Physiotherapy for amputees, —* 'the Roehampton approach.' Churchill Livingstone, Edinburgh

Gordon, T., Castelli, W.P., Hjortland, M.C., Kannel, W.B. and Dawber, T.R. (1977) 'Predicting heart disease in middle-aged and older patients.' *J.A.M.A., 238*, 497

Hadi, O.A., Morris, J. and Kicher, P.H. (1980) 'Care during and after the acute attack.' *Ger. Med. 104*, 46

Katrak, P.H. and Baggot, J.B. (1980) 'Rehabilitation of elderly lower extremity amputees.' *Med. J. Australia,1*, 651-3

McCollough, N.G. (1971) 'The dysvascular amputee. Surgery and rehabilitation.' *Curr. Prob. Surg., 1*

McMillan, J.B. and Lev, M. (1964) 'The ageing heart II: the valves.' *J. Gerontol. 19*, 1-6

Mensch, G. and Ellis, P. (1982) 'Physical therapeutic management of lower limb amputees.' In S.N. Bannerjee (ed), *Rehabilitation management of amputees*, Williams and Wilkins, Baltimore

Montoye, J., Willis, P.W. and Cunningham, D.A. (1968) 'Heart rate and responses to submaximal exercise: relation to age and sex.' *J. Gerontol, 23*, 127

O'Connell, M. (1984) 'A comparative study of pain relief in o.a. knees.' *Abstracts, 5*, 1, 9-13

Parbhoo, S.P. (1979) 'Venous Ulcers.' *Ger. Med., 9*, 6, 60

Robinson, K.P. (1976) 'Long posterior flap amputation in geriatric patients with ischaemic disease.' *Ann. R.C. Surg. Eng. 58*, 440

Rosenham, R.H. (1970) 'Coronary heart disease in the western collaborative study: A follow-up experience of four and a half years.' *J. Chronic Dis. 23*, 173-6

Savage, B. (1960) *Practical electrotherapy for physiotherapists*. Faber and Faber, London

Sjorgren, A.L. (1971) 'Left ventricular wall thickness determined by ultrasound in 100 subjects without chest disease.' *Chest, 60*, 341

Steinberg, F.O., Garcia, W.J. and Rositger, R.F. (1974) 'Rehabilitation of the geriatric amputee.' *J. Ger. Soc. 22*, 62–6

Thould, A.L. (1965) 'Coronary heart disease in the aged.' *Brit. Med. J., 2*, 1089

Wale, J.O. (1961) *Tidy's massage and remedial exercises*. Wright, Bristol

Williams, B.O., Begg, T.B., Semple, T. and McGuiness, J.B. (1976) 'The elderly in a coronary unit.' *Brit. Med. J. 2*, 451–3

8

Disorders of the Respiratory System

Elderly people are susceptible to virtually all of the many respiratory diseases. Older patients who have respiratory diseases develop complications more often than younger patients either because of disease in other organs, or because of a combination of pulmonary problems (Ziment 1982). The major symptom complexes involving the lungs of older patients are infection, obstructive-airways disease and respiratory failure. Malignant neoplasm and pulmonary embolus are also common.

Lung infection declines measurably after maturity because of the ageing process itself, environmental factors such as cigarette-smoking and air pollution and possibly unidentified genetic and metabolic influences. The fall in the forced expiratory volume in one second (FEV_1) with age averages about 25 ml per year. However the fall is not linear and a decrease of approximately 20 ml per year has been recorded in the 25–39 age group, with acceleration in this decrease to 38 ml per year in people aged 65 and over. There is also a decrease in the arterial oxygen tension but the arterial carbon dioxide tension remains the same (Brandstetter and Kazemi 1986). The costal cartilages become more rigid with age, the inspiratory and intercostal muscles are shortened and these changes are often accompanied by some degree of kyphosis. This results in attenuated coughing mechanism and difficulty in clearing secretions from the bronchial tree. Atrophy of the ciliated epithelium compounds the problem.

OBSTRUCTIVE-AIRWAYS DISEASES

Obstructive-airways disease is the major cause of pulmonary

136

disability in the elderly (Wynne 1979). The management of chronic bronchitis, emphysema and asthma forms a major part of a physiotherapist's case load when working with elderly patients.

CHRONIC BRONCHITIS

Chronic bronchitis was defined by the World Health Organization (1961) as the presence of a productive cough for at least three months of the year for more than two consecutive years. The cough results from excessive production of tracheobronchial mucus. Hyperplasia and hypertrophy of the mucous glands in the submucosa of the large airways are often present, while in the small airways, chronic inflammation and oedema, plus increased smooth muscle and goblet-cell hyperplasia may be noted. Smoking is an important factor in the aetiology and many elderly men have been life-long smokers. The typical chronic bronchitic is the 'blue bloater'; overweight, somnolent, oedematous and plethoric patient with polycythaemia, hypoxia and pulmonary hypertension.

Treatment of acute exacerbation

Respiratory infections complicating chronic bronchitis are usually due to *Streptococcus pneumoniae* or to *Haemophilus influenza*. Most infections respond to commonly used antibiotics such as amoxycillin, ampicillin or cotrimoxazole. Whenever possible, especially in a hospital setting, sputum should be obtained for culture and sensitivity before commencing treatment and chest physiotherapy may be necessary to get a good specimen. Oxygen therapy may be required in severe infection but its use should be monitored carefully with estimations of blood gas to avoid carbon dioxide narcosis. It is usual to use a Ventimask 24% and oxygen is delivered through a humidifier in hospital. This prevents drying and discomfort of the upper airways. The traditional use of humidification as a method of increasing mucus clearance has been challenged in recent years as there is little evidence to prove that controlled humidity is either beneficial or harmful. Some claim that the use of water or saline aerosols may work by increasing the effectiveness of coughing and so help mucus clearance. The use of mucolytic agents such as acetylcysteine is even more controversial as clinical trials to assess their value have on the whole been disappointing.

137

Patients who have a persistent and productive cough may require regular postural drainage performed more frequently during exacerbations. Percussion and vibrations may be used to loosen secretions, but in the elderly they must be administered with care and consideration for the patient's overall condition. Most patients tolerate drainage, though a modified form may be required such as lying on alternate sides with the bed elevated 30–45 cm at the foot. In hospital, drainage should be given for at least 30 minutes, twice a day. If a patient is being prescribed bronchodilators, these should be given prior to drainage. Bronchodilators decrease bronchial muscle tone, inhibit release of chemical mediators of asthma from mast cells, improve movement of tracheal mucus and aid in the clearance of secretions from the lung (Wynne 1979). All beta-adrenergic bronchodilators can stimulate the cardiovascular system and in the elderly, caution should be observed. The presence of angina or arrythmia would be considered a contraindication.

Some elderly patients find the technique of using pressurised aerosols difficult and for them the newer 'space inhalers' may be of value. However, some patients find them cumbersome and embarrassing. During an acute exacerbation, bronchodilator therapy may be given by nebuliser.

Bronchial hygiene is greatly dependent upon the effectiveness of the cough mechanism. The ability to take a deep breath is essential for an effective cough and to accomplish the optimum peripheral distribution of inspired air by providing a slow inspiratory pause. Breathing control should be taught and it is customary to teach patients, diaphragmatic breathing and localised expansion of lateral and posterior basal segments of the lung. Evidence suggests that such exercise probably does not achieve the specific objective; however, the value is that the patient is taught a slow, deep-breathing pattern that allows more complete emptying of the lungs and improves alveolar ventilation (Becklake 1954). It will also control the tendency of patients to hyperventilate in response to stress and so avoid increased airway collapse and trapping of air. A patient whose breathing and coughing capabilities are significantly limited may receive benefit from intermittent-positive-pressure-breathing (IPPB). Intermittent-positive-pressure-breathing is the most expensive respiratory-treatment modality commonly used by physiotherapists and although literature of the effect of IPPB is vast, it is also inconclusive (O'Sullivan 1982).

On administration of IPPB, tidal volume must exceed 75% of the limited vital capacity. The treatment should be administered before other forms of treatment and should be supervised. The patient must be instructed very carefully before using IPPB. He must understand why the treatment is being used and what is hoped to be accomplished by it. The routine administration of IPPB is unnecessary and ineffective in the absence of good indications. During an acute-on-chronic attack, it is possible that the patient will go into hypercapnic respiratory failure. This is discussed later in the chapter.

Maintenance treatment

There will be a need for continuing care. Often therapists are inclined to be concerned with the acute exacerbation of the disorder, but neglect the on-going chronic disease. Patients should be advised to avoid the irritants that are known to exacerbate symptoms. For example, dust, cigarette smoke, polluted air, changes in temperature and humidity will all exacerbate symptoms. Common sense is needed when offering advice.

For the chronic phase, the aims are:

1. Maintenance of postural drainage;
2. Maintenance of breathing control;
3. Coping with emergencies;
4. Coping with activities of daily living.

Communication with all patients is essential and the elderly patient must have the reason for maintenance treatment carefully explained. Patients with chronic bronchitis will need to carry out postural drainage at home. It is rarely possible to 'tip' a bed in the same manner as in hospital. The problem may be overcome by giving the patient a roll of newspapers tied together, about 15 cm thick. Pillows are placed over the roll on a firm surface and the patient is shown how to lie over it in a variety of positions.

It is important to encourage patients to maintain the deep-breathing and controlled-breathing exercises that they were shown in hospital. It is helpful if the patient is shown a simple relaxation technique in conjunction with the breathing exercises. Emphasis should not be placed on expiration but on 'getting air in'. Patients will become short of breath from time to time and so it can be stressed that if control of breathing and relaxation are mastered, this will help them in times of stress.

If a patient becomes short of breath, there are five basic positions

Figure 8.1: Forward-lean sitting

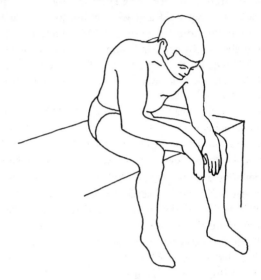

Figure 8.2: Forward-lean standing

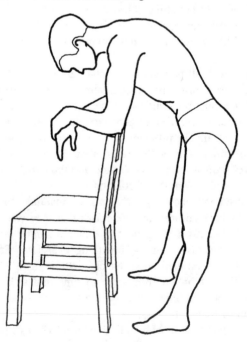

for relaxation and breathing control that they may be shown (Gaskell 1979). These are high side-lying, forward-lean sitting (Fig. 8.1), relaxed sitting, forward-lean standing (Fig. 8.2) and relaxed standing. The common feature of all these positions is that the patient is comfortably supported; the shoulders and arms are relaxed and an overall flexion posture is maintained.'

Elderly patients with chest disease become very distressed when walking upstairs or up hills (even of quite small incline). The aim of treatment is to help them to breathe in a rhythm with their steps. There is little value in being dogmatic and telling a patient to breathe in for two steps and out for one step. One should find the patient's natural rhythm and build on that, encouraging a longer inspiratory effort and concentrating little on expiratory effort. Many patients become distressed if they have to bend down to pick up objects or to do up their shoe laces. Alternative methods have to be found and, where helpful, simple aids provided.

It is of little value to give exercises to increase the mobility of the thorax in the elderly, as deformities will be irreversible, but general exercises will improve tolerance and this will make the necessary daily activities much easier to perform. All patients should be put on a programme of graduated exercise; programmes must be supervised and this demands out-patient attendance. Unless follow-up is continuous, patients will tend to 'give up'. Sedentary habits are not to be condoned in chronic bronchitics.

EMPHYSEMA

Emphysema is defined by the distension of air spaces distal to the terminal bronchiole and destruction of alveolar septa. The elasticity of the lung is lost and it becomes fixed in inspiration so that little gas exchange takes place. Emphysematous changes in the lungs are found in 50 per cent of people over the age of sixty. (Wynne 1979). The typical emphysematous patient is the 'pink puffer' — a thin, undernourished, hyperinflated person struggling to breathe. There are characteristic changes on the chest x-ray with widely spaced ribs, a flat diaphragm, a narrow mediastinal shadow and hyperinflated lung fields. Sputum is scant rather than copious as in chronic bronchitis. Patients with severe emphysema have a very poor prognosis. In many cases of chronic bronchitis, there is co-existent emphysema. The presence of emphysema aggravates the symptoms of chronic bronchitis. Pulmonary hypertension may

141

develop and this in turn may lead to congestive cardiac failure.

Treatment of emphysema

The primary aim of the physiotherapy treatment of emphysema is to teach the patient to breathe with the least effort and in so doing, to encourage a better pattern of breathing in terms understood by the patient. An explanation of the mechanism of breathing should be given and it is also important that the patient can appreciate a 'relaxed' state. The emphasis, as with chronic bronchitis, is on the inspiratory and not the expiratory phase. Grant (1970) in a review of the literature showed that controlled breathing did not significantly improve a patient's pulmonary-function tests. However, in the elderly it is difficult to exclude latent or underlying disease that will affect such tests and patients would seem to derive benefit from the fact that they are breathing in a more economical way. It is interesting to see the relationship between improvement in function (i.e. ability to perform everyday tasks) and the pulmonary-function tests. McGavin *et al.* (1977) found that in an exercise scheme that involved climbing ten steps daily for ten minutes (at least once a day), exercise tolerance as judged by the twelve-minute-walk test increased, whilst ventilatory-function tests remained unchanged.

Patients are often fearful and anxious of their condition and treatment can allay these fears and anxieties. In emphysema, if there are secretions present, then postural drainage may assist their removal. Whenever a physiotherapist treats a patient suffering from a chest disorder, it is an opportunity to give health advice, especially in relation to smoking. In a study on the participation of the elderly in psychological studies Lye (1982) showed that most individuals are impressed by such advice, though he added that he had no way of knowing if the advice was effective.

ASTHMA

Asthma is characterised by hyperactivity of the airways on exposure to various stimuli. Narrowing of the airways results in bronchospasm, bronchial-wall oedema and hypersecretion by mucous glands leading to wheezing and coughing.

The aims of physiotherapy are:

1. To relieve bronchospasm;
2. To encourage relaxation and gain control of breathing;
3. To assist in the removal of secretions;
4. To improve the pattern of breathing.

(Webber 1980)

Until such time as bronchospasm is relieved, it will be impossible to mobilise the secretions. In the elderly especially, any attempt to remove secretions whether by coughing or postural drainage prior to bronchodilation will be on the one hand tiring and on the other, may well induce or aggravate bronchospasm. Bronchodilators are given with care to the elderly because as stated earlier, beta-adrenergic dilators can stimulate the cardiovascular system. Intravenous aminophylline and steroids may be used to induce bronchodilation in a severe attack.

Simple lung-function tests may be carried out (Wright's Peak Flow) before and after administration of treatment to assess response. The bronchodilator may be given either by metered dose inhaler, a nebuliser or an intermittent positive pressure breathing device. There is no evidence to show that bronchodilator solutions inhaled from a simple nebuliser by mouthpiece are inferior to intermittent positive pressure breathing (Webber, Shenfield and Paterson 1974). The patient should be well-supported in a relaxed position and inhale using diaphragmatic breathing. Relaxation and control of breathing are very important to the asthmatic. The patient is shown the relaxed positions mentioned earlier, which are well described in many physiotherapy texts (Gaskell 1979 and Webber 1980). In these positions, the patient is encouraged to breathe gently, with emphasis on slowing down the rate. It will be noted that patients use accessory muscles of respiration and have difficulty in achieving an adequate expiration phase. Stress is laid on relaxation of the upper chest and use of the lower lateral basal part of the chest. Emphasis is placed on encouragement of expiration, and little made of inspiration. If a patient finds it difficult to expectorate, wait. Do not stress the patient and run the risk of aggravating bronchospasm, but allow time for adequate bronchodilation to take place. When the patient begins to cough and expectorate sputum, encouragement is given and depending upon the patient, modified postural drainage may be attempted. If the patient becomes breathless, or experiences difficulty in expectoration, stop and allow the patient to resume a normal position. Never hurry or put stress on the patient. Pryor and Webber (1979) have demonstrated that forced expiration to produce a cough does not increase bronchospasm.

In the elderly, wheezing is often continuous; exposure to dust, cigarette smoke and so on may well aggravate the patient. Certain elderly patients with asthma show characteristics of both intrinsic and extrinsic disease. Sodium cromoglycate (Intal) helps prevent attacks in patients who are hypersensitive to allergens. It is not as effective in elderly patients as in younger patients, but there are exceptions. Maintenance of low-dose corticosteroid therapy may be necessary in some older patients with persistent problems. If it can be given as an aerosol, significant systemic side effects will be avoided.

RESPIRATORY FAILURE

As the lungs are designed for gas exchange (oxygen repletion and carbon dioxide elimination), respiratory failure is defined in terms of abnormal gas tensions. If the arterial pO_2 is less than 60 mmHG (8.0 kPa) as a consequence of lung disease, the patient is in respiratory failure. A low pO_2 with a normal or low pCO_2 (below 50 mmHg; 6.7 kPa) is described as Type I respiratory failure. The combination of a low pO_2 and an elevated pCO_2 is described as Type II respiratory failure.

Type I

Variations in ventilation/perfusion ratios between different alveoli in the lung are the most frequent cause of Type I failure. Conditions that give rise to impairment of gas exchange in a sufficient number of alveoli will cause this type of failure. It may be found in patients with chronic bronchitis and emphysema before they go on to develop hypercapnia and Type II failure. Other causes include pneumonia, acute pulmonary oedema, pulmonary embolism, asthma and fibrosing alveolitis. High concentrations of inspired oxygen are used in the treatment of Type I respiratory failure.

Type II

Normally hypercapnia produces an increased respiratory drive, but in patients with Type II failure, this mechanism has failed. Type II failure therefore results from problems both in the lung and in the

144

brain centres controlling respiration. It is seen most commonly in elderly patients during an acute exacerbation of chronic bronchitis and emphysema. It may also be seen in patients with severe asthma. Oxygen therapy must be carefully controlled as mentioned earlier when discussing the treatment of acute exacerbation of chronic bronchitis. The patient's respiratory drive is dependent upon hypoxaemia, so that uncontrolled oxygen therapy may actually depress respiratory rate. This would result in a further rise of the arterial pCO_2 leading to respiratory acidosis and possibly the death of the patient. The patient must be encouraged to take deep breaths and to cough and he must be aided to remove secretions. Respiratory stimulants such as doxapram may be used to provide sustained ventilatory stimulation. Mechanical ventilation may be indicated in patients who are failing to respond to a conservative approach. This is often a difficult decision for the physician as some patients have such severe underlying respiratory disease, that it is unlikely that they could be successfully weaned from the ventilator after the acute illness is over. However, in this situation, it is important to stress that it is the patient's respiratory status rather than his or her age that should be the main determining factor in making a decision.

Elderly patients in intensive care units

Elderly patients are likely to have existing chronic disease in other systems which may increase morbidity and mortality in acute respiratory failure. Wilson (1972) has shown that the elderly are prone to intensive-therapy-unit psychosis because of their illness and unusual surroundings. Everything possible should be done to help orientate the patient in relation to personnel and surroundings.

High-risk patients for surgery must have pre-operative instruction and rigorous post-operative care (Lorhan 1971). They are prone to aspiration of food and gastric contents and to the development of pulmonary emboli. It is important that secretions are removed frequently by tracheal suction. Physical restraints are avoided whenever possible; if they are necessary, they must never be positioned so that they restrict chest movement and encourage hypoventilation. Post-operative management will include ventilator care, breathing exercises and postural drainage with vibration and shaking. Particular care must be taken to avoid decubitus ulcers in elderly patients who are critically ill.

BRONCHIECTASIS

Bronchiectasis is an irreversible, abnormal dilation of the bronchi. It may be isolated in specific lung segments, or may affect the whole lung. Bronchopneumonia is now a common cause of bronchiectasis. Classic symptoms are cough, copious sputum and recurrent pneumonia.

The aim of physiotherapy is to assist the patient in the removal of secretions. The patient is shown postural drainage positions that may have to be modified for the individual. A relative or friend is shown how to help the patient manage these positions at home. The physiotherapist should be aware that in some patients, haemoptysis is a common symptom and may be the sole symptom in dry bronchiectasis. In these patients, postural drainage should not be given as it tends to aggravate haemoptysis.

PNEUMONIA

The elderly are more susceptible to and less tolerant of pulmonary infection than younger people. The primary factors are the physiological effects of ageing on the lung, the frequent presence of associated disease and the probable decline of the immune response (Makinodan 1976).

Aspiration of pharyngeal contents into the lung is probably not uncommon in the elderly and is, of course, a major problem with disorders of swallowing. In these secondary pneumonias, bacterial infection may be less important than the stasis of secretions and antibacterial therapy is disappointing in the absence of effective expectoration. Primary pneumonia in those who are normally in good health is most commonly due to *Streptococcus pneumoniae* or *Haemophilus influenzae* but *Staphylococcus aureus* becomes important during epidemics of influenza. Less commonly, a gram-negative organism such as *Klebsiella pneumoniae* or *Pseudomonas aeruginosa* is responsible, especially for pneumonia in hospital.

Pneumonia in the elderly often presents in an atypical fashion. The usual signs of pneumonia such as cough, purulent sputum, fever and pleuritic pain are often absent or mild in the elderly and are replaced by lethargy, loss of appetite, tachypnoea and tachycardia. The cough is frequently unobtrusive.

The treatment of pneumonia in the elderly must include rehydration and adequate oxygenation. The patient should be encouraged to cough and to clear secretions. A Swedish study has challenged the role of chest physiotherapy in primary infectious pneumonia, particularly in younger age groups (Britton, Bejstedt and Vedin 1985). However, patients with chronic bronchitis, emphysema and asthma were excluded from their study. In patients with chronic bronchitis producing copious sputum, conventional chest physiotherapy has been shown to have a beneficial effect on air conductance. It is reasonable to assume that such patients with pneumonia would benefit from chest physiotherapy. Most elderly patients with bronchopneumonia will have secretions from the early stages and vigorous treatment is necessary immediately. Postural drainage with vibrations and shaking is performed. As the patient recovers, he should be shown localised breathing activity as in the section on chronic bronchitis. It is open to question whether bed rest is of benefit and the patient who is not extremely ill should remain mobile to avoid further tendency to develop deep-vein thrombosis.

PULMONARY TUBERCULOSIS

Although antituberculous drugs and improved social conditions have changed the incidence of tuberculosis dramatically in recent decades, the disease is still seen in elderly patients. It is almost always due to re-activation of a lesion that has been dormant for years. Changes in immunity, deteriorating general health and poor social conditions are factors that probably favour re-activation. Some patients may be on long-term steroid therapy. Haemoptysis, cough, dyspnoea, debility and weight-loss are all presenting features. Unless there is a high index of suspicion, the condition is easily missed in the elderly and many cases are undiagnosed at post mortem.

Chest x-ray and sputum examination for acid-fast bacilli are essential investigations. If a suitable specimen of sputum cannot be obtained, a laryngeal swab or early morning gastric lavage may be necessary. The results of therapy with the appropriate agents are excellent, but elderly patients must be followed up carefully after discharge to ensure compliance with the drug regime.

BRONCHIAL CARCINOMA AND CARCINOMA OF THE LUNG

Carcinoma of the lung is now the most common fatal malignancy in men. The outlook for the patient is dismal; the overall five-year survival rate is 5 per cent (Beattie 1974). Associated disease often makes the elderly person with lung cancer a poor candidate for surgery. Carcinoma of the bronchus is the most common tumour in the lung. The diagnosis is often delayed in the older patient because symptoms are assigned to old age rather than medical illness. Cough and shortness of breath may be uncritically attributed to bronchitis or heart failure; pain and haemoptysis lead to earlier diagnosis. Occasionally, an audible wheeze localised to one side may be heard in those complaining of shortness of breath, suggesting occlusion of a major airway by tumour, or there may be evidence of metastatic disease such as lymphadenopathy or hepatomegaly. Frequently however, there are no helpful clinical signs. If clinical evidence suggests a tumour but malignant cells are not found in the sputum, a decision must be made about further investigation. Fibre-optic bronchoscopy is a relatively safe procedure in the elderly.

Surgery is still the treatment of choice for bronchial carcinoma, except in the case of an oat cell tumour. The risk of surgery does not increase with age and pneumonectomy carries a mortality of 15 per cent (Bates 1970). Most elderly patients will prove to be unsuitable for surgery. Half will have disease that is too extensive locally and another quarter will be found to have distant spread or to be unfit for operation (Stark and Dent 1985). The decision to operate or not must also take account of general health, state of mind and home and family circumstances. Whichever form of medical or surgical treatment is decided upon, skilful use of analgesic drugs, as well as care of the well-being of the patient, remain all important.

Physiotherapy

Physiotherapy may be requested for patients with carcinoma of the lung to aid in the removal of secretions. Vigorous treatment is contraindicated because of the risk of haemoptysis and the likelihood of metastases in the ribs, which could fracture.

CHEST PAIN

The causes of chest pain in the elderly are little different from those of other age groups, but an accurate history may be more difficult to obtain. The cause of localised chest pain (not cardiac, oesophageal, or spinal) can usually be discovered by careful history and clinical assessment. Pleuritic pain may signal severe underlying disease. An infective cause of acute pleurisy is rare unless associated with pneumonia, in which case the features of pneumonia will be evident. Thrombo-embolism is an important cause of pleuritic pain. Acute pleuritic pain is not a common initial manifestation of cancer or tuberculosis in the elderly.

Pain from the ribs or from soft tissue of the chest wall can mimic pleurisy. Both may be worse on inspiration and movement, but marked local tenderness suggests a chest-wall rather than pleural source and pain from the chest wall can usually be reproduced exactly by firm pressure over one spot on the chest, either over a rib or a costo-sternal joint. The severe burning pain that precedes the eruption of zoster (See Chapter 9) may cause temporary diagnostic difficulty, but there may be hyperaesthesia over the area. The pain of malignant deposits in the ribs or of direct involvement of the chest wall by tumour is more persistent and constant and local swelling or tenderness may be found.

REFERENCES

Bates, M. (1970) 'Results of surgery for bronchial carcinoma in patients aged 70 and over.' *Thorax*, *25*, 77–8

Beattie, E.J. (1970) 'Operative mortality and five-year-survival rates in men with bronchogenic carcinoma.' *Chest*, *66*, 469–74

Becklake, M.R. (1954) 'A study of the effects of physiotherapy in chronic hypertrophic emphysema using lung function tests.' *Dis. Chest.*, *26*, 180–5

Brandstetter, R.D. and Kazemi, H. (1986) 'Ageing and the respiratory system.' *Med. Clinics of N. America*

Britton, S., Bejstedt, M. and Vedin, L. (1985) 'Chest physiotherapy in primary pneumonia.' *Brit. Med. J.*, *290*, 1703–4

Gaskell, D.V. (1979) 'An introduction to medical chest conditions.' In P.A. Downie (ed), *Cash's textbook of chest, heart and vascular diseases for physiotherapists*, 2nd edn, Faber and Faber, London

Grant, R. (1970) 'The physiological basis for increased exercise ability in patients with emphysema after breathing exercise training.' *Physiotherapy*, *55*, 12, 541–7

Lye, M. (1982) 'Will the elderly participate in physiological studies?' *Resp. News. Bull.* *24*, 2, 10–14

Lorhan, P.H. (1971) *Anaesthesia in the Aged*. Charles C. Thomas, Springfield, Illinois

McGavin, C.R., Gupta, S.P., Lloyd, E.C. and McHardy, G.J.R. (1977) 'The physical rehabilitation for the chronic bronchitic: results of a controlled trial in the home.' *Thorax*, *32*, 307–10

Makinodan, T. (1976) 'Immunology of ageing.' *J. Am. Geriat. Soc., 24*, 249–54

O'Sullivan, A.P. (1982) 'Intermittent positive pressure breathing', Project submitted, University of Dublin

Pryor, J.A. and Webber, B.A. (1979) 'An evaluation of the forced expiratory technique as an adjunct to postural drainage.' *Physiotherapy, 65*, 10, 304–7

Stark, J.E. and Dent, R.G. (1985) 'Chest diseases.' In A.N. Exton-Smith and M.E. Weksler (eds), *Practical geriatric medicine*, Churchill Livingstone, Edinburgh

Webber, B.A., Shenfield, G.M. and Paterson, J.W. (1974) 'A comparison of three different techniques for giving nebulised albuterol to asthmatic patients.' *Am. Rev. of Resp. Dis., 109*, 293–9

——— (1980) *The Brompton guide to chest physiotherapy.* Blackwell Scientific, Oxford

Wilson, L.M. (1972) 'Intensive care delirium.' *Arch. Int. Med., 130*, 225–30

World Health Organization (1961) 'Definition and diagnosis of pulmonary disease with special reference to chronic bronchitis and emphysema.' *WHO technical report series, 213*, 15

Wynne, J.W. (1979) 'Pulmonary disease in the elderly.' In I. Rossman (ed), *Clinical geriatrics*, Lippincott, Philadelphia

Ziment, I. (1982) 'Management of respiratory problems in the aged.' *Suppl. J. Am. Geriat. Assoc. 30*, 11S, 536–41

9

Skin and Pressure Sores

The biological changes that take place in the skin with ageing have already been outlined in Chapter 1. Skin conditions that involve physiotherapy treatments are described in this chapter.

PSORIASIS

Psoriasis affects all age groups. The typical lesion of psoriasis is papular and covered with fine silver-like scales. The scales, when removed, reveal bleeding points. The main areas to be affected are the extensor surfaces, elbows, knees and low back. The nails are typically affected, the earliest change being pitting on the surface of the nails.

Treatment of psoriasis is not easy. However, it has long been known that the beneficial effect of sunlight is enhanced by coal-tar preparations. The patient is given a coal-tar bath and the skin 'scrubbed' free from as many scales as possible. This is followed by a sub-erythemal dose of ultraviolet irradiation daily. Care must be taken to prepare a test dose after the patient has had a tar bath, as tar acts as a sensitiser. Sometimes an E3 ultraviolet irradiation is given locally to severely affected areas; this dose is given weekly. The scaly area is then coated with tar ointment and covered with stockinette. If involvement is severe, photochemotherapy may be used (Knight 1979). Psoralen medications are combined with long-wave ultraviolet (UVA) in PUVA treatment. However, there is a risk in the long term of skin carcinoma, but whether this is of relevance in the elderly is debatable.

HERPES ZOSTER

Herpes zoster is caused by the varicella-zoster virus. The hallmarks are severe pain and the appearance of a vesicular eruption, which follows a dermatomal distribution. Depending on the location and severity, this condition can be quite incapacitating and devastating.

The disease itself is usually self-limiting and treatment has two aspects, firstly, the care of the vesicular eruption until it heals spontaneously and secondly, the treatment of pain. Pain may be severe and may persist long after the eruption has cleared. This is often true in the older patient, especially if the person is depressed. Ultrasonic treatment (0.3 Wcm^{-3}) has been shown to relieve pain, particularly with trigeminal nerve involvement (O'Beirne 1982). Laser therapy, using an IR CEB laser with three-minute applications along the course of the nerve, has given promising results. Ultraviolet irradiation with an E3 may be used as a counter-irritant. Interferential (90–100 Hz) or ultra-Reiz also give a patient temporary relief of pain.

BURNS

Two age groups are especially vulnerable to burns, the very young and the elderly (Hummel 1982). In a study on 'Age Differences in the Severity and Outcome of Burn', Linn (1980) showed that the death rate for elderly burn patients was four times that of any other group. The same study also demonstrated that elderly persons suffer more severe burns. More often than not, the elderly either live alone or with an elderly partner. An underlying medical condition is often the cause or a contributory cause of an accident.

Prevention

Older people are most frequently involved in fires between 7.00 and 10.00 a.m. It is believed that this is because they tend to be at their least alert when they rise in the morning. Early morning fire and burn accidents could be minimised by purchase of flame retardant sleepwear, not smoking in the early morning, being sure to turn off the gas between the first and second matches and avoiding hazardous tasks until later in the day.

Smoking is a major cause of fire and burn deaths among older people. The highest risk situation is referred to by the fire service as the 'fatal triangle'. The triangle is comprised of a cigarette smoked in an overstuffed chair by a person who is tired or under stress and/or under the influence of alcohol or drugs.

The elderly should, whenever possible, select flame-retardant clothing. They need to know that some fibres such as wool, acrylic, polyester or nylon are more difficult to ignite and burn more slowly than most untreated cottons and polyester/ cotton blends. The elderly should be reminded that, when they are cooking, loose-fitting clothing such as dressing gowns with wide sleeves can be hazardous.

Older people should remove burning clothes or wrap themselves in a blanket as quickly as possible. Due to other health problems, older people are more likely to succumb to smoke inhalation than younger people and may not be able to escape via some routes. They should be advised of suitable escape routes and should practise using these. They should know how to minimise the amount of smoke inhaled by staying low, placing a wet cloth over the mouth and nose and stuffing a rag or towel under a door while waiting for help. ·

Many people find themselves living alone for the first time in old age. This is especially true of women, who because of longer life-expectancy are often left alone or in unfamiliar surroundings late in life. Almost all older people lose someone whom they have depended on, whether for company, meals or small household repairs and errands. These people have to deal with a sense of loss and grief and learn new skills at the same time. Fire-safety information should include household 'hints' such as the proper lighting of pilot lights, how to check and change fuses, how to use and maintain heating units and how to call the fire authority for information and help.

Practice is an essential ingredient of teaching fire-safety measures. Older people should be taught the importance of emptying ashtrays into the fireplace, the placing of a sparkguard in front of the fire and the switching off and unplugging of appliances, especially the television, when not in use. Fire safety should form an important part of the assessment during all home visits. The elderly are less likely to be able to afford investment in fire extinguishers, escape ladders, smoke detectors or the replacement of faulty appliances.

Rehabilitation of the burns patient

Rehabilitation of the burns patient begins on the day of admission. The physiotherapist must anticipate potential impairment during the acute phase and include prophylactic measures during the early treatment regime to prevent deformities and disability. The overall goal of the physical treatment is to restore optimal function to the burns patient as quickly as possible.

Prevention of cross-infection

Contamination of a burn can be caused by self-infection and cross-infection. The physiotherapist is in intimate contact with the patient and the chances of cross-infection are considerable

Respiratory care and prevention of chest complications

About 80 per cent of people sustaining severe burns develop chest complications, especially if the burn involves the face, neck and chest. There may be difficulty in coughing due to the injury, oedema and weakness. This requires postural drainage with general chest care, percussion, vibrations and suctioning to remove excessive secretions. Postural drainage is contraindicated with facial and laryngeal oedema, as it would tend to increase the oedema.

After grafting operations, percussion over the grafted areas should be avoided. Bulky dressings around the chest and abdomen may restrict breathing and this must be counteracted by breathing exercises. It is necessary to monitor the general mobility of elderly patients, as immobility may lead to hypostatic pneumonia.

Prevention of contractures

Careful positioning of all burned parts of the body is essential during hospitalisation. The purpose of positioning is to counteract the tendency of burned areas to develop skin, muscle and joint contractures due to scarring.

The elderly do not normally have much medial rotation of their lower limbs, consequently the hips tend to roll passively into lateral

Table 9.1: Policy for positioning burn patients

Neck	Towel roll or hyperextension mattress No pillows for anterior burns.
Shoulders	Axillary burns require 90° abduction and lateral rotation Patients are removed from braces or slings only for activity, meals and dressing.
Elbows	Full extension If burns are posterior only — some flexion.
Hands	Safe position of up to 35° wrist extension; 70° flexion at metacarpophalangeal joints; extension at proximal and distal interphalangeal joints Thumb in adduction and opposition; no hyperextension at distal interphalangeal joint.
Knees	Position in full extension If burns are anterior only — some flexion.
Hips	15°–30° abduction for burns on the medial aspect of the thigh Extension at the hip joint.
Feet	Neutral position.

Source: Hummel 1982

rotation; this may cause common peroneal nerve compression.

Exercise

Activity is an essential part of the treatment of a burns patient. It assists in the prevention of contractures and minimises oedema. It also prevents loss of power and preserves muscle and vascular tone. Toe, foot and ankle exercises help prevent deep-vein thrombosis.

In the early stages, a patient should be treated three to four times a day. Poorly motivated patients require constant encouragement to perform their exercises. The patient should be encouraged to perform the exercises at least six times a day on their own. Passive exercise increases the possibility of causing microtears in an already damaged and inelastic tissue. This subsequently increases scar formation. Mobilisation of a painful, stiff joint should be co-ordinated with dressing changes; this both minimises the time of discomfort for the patient and enables the physiotherapist to observe any spontaneous rupture. Gentle, gradual movements are preferred to fast, forceful movements. Following grafting, active exercise to the grafted zone is discontinued for three to ten days. During the time of immobilisation, the patient is shown isometric exercises for the involved part in order to maintain muscle tone and increase the circulation.

Splinting

Splinting can help maintain good, functional joint-positioning and prevent serious deformities. There are a number of thermoplastic materials available. These are suitable as they can be moulded easily and repeatedly on the patient.

Hydrotherapy

Hydrotherapy is being used in the treatment of burns. Immersion in a Hubbard tank ensures that all parts of the burn will be exposed and covered by bacteriocidal disinfectant. It has been shown that numbers of bacteria can be reduced using a suitable disinfectant (Smith *et al.* 1975; Bohannon 1982). Promotion of tissue growth is important; granulation tissue and epithelialisation are stimulated by hydrotherapy.

Discharge

Home circumstances will dictate the time of discharge. The physiotherapist will have to work closely with the medical social worker. The medical social worker will deal with the practical problems regarding home and family and on discharge, will make arrangements for any supportive measures that may be necessary.

The patient and the family will be instructed and checked on all exercises, the use of splints, pressure garments and activities of daily living. Follow-up treatment is necessary if contractures are to be avoided. This may best be carried out at a centre near to the patient's home.

PRESSURE SORES

Pressure sores are found most commonly over bony prominences. Unrelieved pressure is by far the most important factor in the causation of deep pressure sores. Tissue anoxia occurs when the capillary blood flow is occluded. Tissue inflammation is another important factor and this is particularly likely to occur when a patient lying in a semi-recumbent position is allowed to slide forward in bed. Patient immobility is the most common cause of unrelieved pressure and patients who are acutely ill are particularly at risk. Contrary to popular belief, pressure sores are not a problem in properly run extended-care wards. In the acutely ill patient, many of the systemic factors such as impaired circulation, dehydration and pyrexia reduce the resistance of tissue to damage and predispose the patient to developing pressure sores. Pressure sores can be prevented by identifying patients who are at risk on admission and by insuring that these patients are turned regularly. Early mobilisation of acutely ill patients is also important and it must be remembered that patients who are sitting at their bedside should be mobilised regularly (Barbenel et al. 1977). Pressures are very high on supporting tissues when the patient is seated.

There are a great many special devices which are available for the prevention of pressure sores. Broadly speaking, they can be divided into two groups. Those that reduce the length of time a particular site is exposed to high pressure and those that reduce the magnitude of pressure acting on the site by re-distributing the weight over a wider area. Examples of the former group would be an alternating pressure mattress and a constantly tilting bed. The water bed, the net-suspension bed and bead-pillow mattresses are examples of the second group. The danger of using special beds like these is that too much reliance might be placed on them. For instance, if there is a water bed on the ward, it is tempting to put an immobile patient into it rather than having to turn the patient regularly. This tends to shift responsibility for preventing pressure sores away from the staff and on to the water bed. However, the use of special beds is not without hazard. For instance, to place a Parkinson's patient with a chest infection in a water bed may lead to the patient's death. He will become more immobile in the bed and this will not benefit his Parkinson's disease or his chest problem. A net-suspension bed, which is essentially a nylon mesh net supported on two horizontal poles above the bed, can also impede chest movement. The correct course of action therefore depends on the individual case and

157

appropriate members of the team should be consulted before making the decision (Coakley and Hu 1982).

Sheepskin is commonly used as a comfortable support, either to lie on or to sit on and natural sheepskin is an excellent interface material. A number of pads have been designed to prevent pressure sores. These include cushions filled with expanded polystyrene, synthetic-gel cushions and water cushions. Rubber rings should not be used as they increase local oedema due to venous stasis and they obstruct arterial supply to the area. Coakley and Rhodes (1982) describe a pad that is attached to the patient and is designed to give protection during acute illness.

Treatment of established pressure sores

Deep pressure sores are treated by the removal of tissue and the cleaning of the ulcer base. Slough may be removed by surgical debridement or by de-sloughing agents. There are numerous de-sloughing agents available such as enzyme preparations, hydrophilic microscopic beads and various creams. All of these have their advocates and some are very expensive. At present, calcium hypochloride solution (Eusol) is probably used most widely for de-sloughing sores. There is also a wide choice of dressings available including soft polyester foam dressings and silicone foam elastomer dressings.

Heterograft skin (porcine dermis) has been used as a temporary dressing. There are many synthetic biological dressings available. Plastic surgery can diminish the prolonged period that is often necessary to heal a pressure sore by conservative methods. The ulcer must be clean and granulating before surgery. The wide range of treatments can be very confusing. It is advisable that the team should become familiar with one sensible treatment regime rather than switch regularly to the newest 'wonder cure' on the market.

Oxygen under ambient pressure may exert a healing effect but it is suggested that hyperbaric oxygen is more effective. It sterilises the wound and enhances granulation and epithelium formation (Fisher 1969). Ionozone treatment is a more recent development. It consists of ionised water, ozone and oxygen and is produced by passing steam over a mercury vapour arc. It appears to be particularly good for pain relief (Dolphin and Walker 1979).

Physiotherapy care of pressure sores

Ultraviolet irradiation

This is one of the traditional methods of treating a pressure sore, particularly when sores are infected and sloughing. The treatment may be divided into two. Firstly, the treatment of the skin surrounding the sore to improve circulation and secondly, the treatment of the sore cavity.

There are differences of opinion concerning the most suitable erythema dosage. For the surrounding skin, the most common application is an E1, which helps to improve the condition of the skin and stimulates circulation. The most common dose for the cavity is an E4 (2), to cause a sloughing of necrotic tissue. The frequency of application of the ultraviolet causes even greater controversy than the dosage level. However, consensus shows that the E1 may be repeated daily, but that the E4 (2) should be given no more frequently than on alternate days. Clinical trials are required to clarify treatment in this area.

Ultrasonics

Where the wound is particularly deep, this technique is a useful alternative to ultraviolet irradiation. The dosage used is 0.5 Wcm^{-2}, pulsed at 1:4. The most suitable frequency is 3 MHz, used for three to five minutes active-treatment time. The skin is washed with Savlon prior to treatment and the transducer head is soaked in Savlon after use. The sore itself is not treated, but insonation is given to the surrounding area.

REFERENCES

Barbenal, J.C., Jordan, M.M., Nicol, S.M. and Clarke, M.O. (1977) 'Instance of pressure sores in the Greater Glasgow Health Board Area.' *Lancet, ii*, 2548

Bohannon, R.W. (1982) 'Whirlpool versus whirlpool and rinse for removal of bacteria from venous stasis ulcer.' *J. Am. Phys. Ther. Assoc., 62*, 304–7

Coakley, D. and Rhodes, J. (1982) 'Pressure sores. a new approach to prevention.' *Geriatric Med, 12*, 3, 54–5

Coakley, D. and Hu, J. (1982) 'Pressure sores — a shared responsibility.' In D. Coakley and V.J. Hanson (eds), *Nursing and the Doctor*, Pitman Medical, London

Dolphin, S. and Walker, M. (1979) 'Healing accelerated by ionozone therapy.' *Physiotherapy, 65*, 3, 81–3

Fisher, B.H. (1969) 'Topical hyperbaric oxygen treatment of pressure sores and skin ulcers.' *Lancet, ii*, 405–8

Hummel, R.P. (1982) *Clinical burn therapy — management and prevention*. Wright, Bristol

Knight, A.G. (1979) 'PUVA therapy for mycosis fungicides.' *Geriatric Med., 9*, 62

Linn, B.S. (1980) 'Age differences in the severity and outcome of burns.' *J. Am. Ger. Soc., 28*, 118–23

O'Beirne, M. (1982) 'Herpes zoster and ultrasound.' *Abstracts, 3* 3, 9

Smith, R., Blasi, D., Dayton, S. and Chipps, D. (1974) 'Effects of sodium hypochlorite on the microbial flora of burns and normal skin.' *J. of Trauma*, 938–41

10

Psychiatry of Elderly Patients

Psychogeriatrics, like psychiatry in general, has been a somewhat neglected area in the syllabus of schools of physiotherapy. Yet nearly a quarter of those patients admitted to psychiatric units are over 65 and suffer from the same physical problems of ageing as those admitted or cared for in other areas of the health services. Likewise, many elderly patients admitted to medical, surgical and geriatric wards may have a psychiatric problem as well as physical disabilities. If physiotherapists are to treat these patients in a meaningful way, they must have some understanding of the psychiatric conditions with which they are confronted.

Several community surveys have indicated that between 20 and 25 per cent of the population over 65 years old suffer from identifiable psychiatric disability. Most attention has been focused on the problem of severe dementia, which affects about 5 per cent of this population. However, the majority of elderly people with psychiatric disability are suffering from conditions such as mild dementia, depression, anxiety or personality disorders. Very few patients with psychiatric morbidity in old age receive treatment for the condition. This is probably due to the fact that illness in older people, whether mental or physical, is all too readily attributed to ageing. It may also be dismissed as simply a reaction to social deprivation. Moreover, elderly people with psychiatric problems tend to become withdrawn and are therefore unlikely to ask for help.

There is a gradual decline in perceptual and motor functions with increasing age. These changes are thought to be due both to deterioration in peripheral sensory mechanisms and to degenerative changes in the brain. The brain is less efficient at storing new information so short-term memory becomes impaired. It is also less efficient at learning new concepts or at handling unfamiliar relationships. In normal ageing, intellectual decline and deterioration of memory occur very slowly and in an orderly progression, whereas in pathological conditions, changes occur rapidly and irregularly (Post 1978). As a result of these intellectual changes the older person becomes less receptive to new ideas and prefers routine. This makes it more difficult for them to cope with stress whether physical or mental.

The increase in the number of elderly people in the community has paradoxically been accompanied by several changes in the environment that make life more difficult for them. The trappings of modern society such as supermarkets, fast cars and bureaucracy all generate tension. Shopping in a modern city is an adventure full of risk for an old person with diminished sight and hearing. Many elderly people in inner-city areas are very isolated and they live in fear of vandalism and burglary (Coakley and Woodford Williams 1979). This has an adverse effect on their health. Events that give rise to increased stress are associated with the onset of a spectrum of medical, surgical and psychiatric illness. Situations that provoke feelings of hopelessness are particularly likely to lead to ill health.

SELF-NEGLECT

Some elderly people live at home in conditions that most people would consider appalling. An unkempt old person living in a very dirty and untidy house may alarm neighbours or visiting therapists. However, before any hasty decisions are made, it is important to establish whether the old person is not coping or whether it is just a question of eccentricity. Some people appear to reject society's standards of cleanliness and opt to live in squalor. They may collect large quantities of specific items such as tinned food in the house. Many people who neglect themselves like this in old age have had responsible jobs in society. The condition is sometimes known as Diogenes' syndrome after the famous ancient cynic who never washed and who eventually lived in a large earthenware jar. There is often pressure to institutionalise people who live in squalor. This, however, should never be a first option as those who live quite happily in chaos may deteriorate rapidly in an institutional environment.

ALCOHOLISM

Despite heavy drinking, some alcoholics survive into old age. They usually have symptoms and physical signs secondary to the prolonged alcohol abuse. They may be ataxic and confused because of damage to the nervous system or there may be signs of liver or cardiac impairment. In recent years, there has been an increasing awareness of alcoholism presenting for the first time in old age. A high index of suspicion is necessary because the patients frequently do not volunteer the information and they may even deny it if questioned directly. Relatives may be unaware of the situation or they may also be reluctant to speak about the problem. Those who indulge in excessive alcohol for the first time in old age are more likely to do so because of environmental stress or illness rather than because of personality problems. Most elderly alcoholics are women and they are particularly susceptible to the damage to the central nervous system associated with excess alcohol intake (Droller 1964).

ANXIETY

Studies in the community suggest that there is a high incidence of neurotic states in the elderly. Bergmann (1979) found that 9 per cent of the elderly were suffering from anxiety states. Anxiety is a normal healthy reaction in situations of stress. It prepares the body for action. However, anxiety is pathological when it begins to pervade the mental life of the elderly person. The person becomes irritable, agitated, forgetful and concentration is impaired. Sleep is disturbed and the appetite is poor. In this situation, anxiety inhibits rather than stimulates the individual. Some elderly patients with anxiety may develop phobias such as agoraphobia (fear of open space).

In the elderly, the onset of a neurosis may follow a physical illness. The illness probably unmasks an underlying insecurity in the patient's personality. On the other hand, anxiety is likely to present with somatic symptoms in the elderly more than in any other age group. These may be hypochondriacal complaints of headaches, palpitations, muscle weakness and similar symptoms. Obsessional/compulsive states may be particularly distressing in old age and they usually occur in people with a life-long history of obsessional tendencies.

Neurosis may be treated by psychotherapy, behavioural therapy, minor tranquillisers and social support, either alone or in combination depending on individual circumstances.

DEPRESSION

In-patient and case-register statistics suggest that the incidence of depression falls in old age. However, this may mean that much depression remains undiagnosed in this age group. In studies of symptoms (as opposed to psychiatrists' diagnosis) it is generally agreed that the highest rates of depressive symptoms are found in the elderly. In a study in Newcastle-upon-Tyne of randomly selected old people living at home, Kay and Beamish (1964) found an incidence of 14 per cent of symptoms of anxiety and disturbance of mood severe enough to cause some interference with activities of daily life. Although physical illness and some drugs can cause depression, the most common cause in the elderly is psychological stress. The various losses that occur in old age such as loss of status, income, health, company and independence may all precipitate depression. Bereavement is the greatest stress and there is an increase in death rate among widowers during the first six months after the death of a spouse.

Symptoms of depression in the elderly include loss of confidence and drive, insomnia, anorexia and weight loss. They may be apathetic and withdrawn or hostile and agitated. The possibility of an underlying depression should always be considered by the physiotherapist when a patient is not co-operating with therapy or not making expected progress. Treatment of the depression is usually successful and modern anti-depressant drugs are very effective. Empathy and an attempt to see their depression as the outcome of a human problem usually helps the patient. Treating any relevant physical disabilities will also facilitate recovery.

MANIA

The manic patient is in a state of pathological exaltation. He is constantly on the move and he sleeps very little. He is full of new ideas and suggestions and he tries to put them all into action at once. He talks non-stop and he can be the life and soul of any group unless thwarted, when he may become aggressive. His mania may also be punctuated by episodes of severe depression. Most elderly people with mania have suffered from the condition in earlier adult life but it can occur for the first time in old age. It is far less common than depression. About 5 per cent of admissions to a general psychogeriatric ward suffer from mania, whereas nearly 50 per cent suffer from depression (Pitt 1982).

A manic episode usually lasts about six weeks. The symptoms may be alleviated by the use of tranquillisers. Lithium carbonate is also used in treatment and to reduce the frequency of recurrences. The manic patient may be difficult for a therapist to cope with because of his hyperactivity. He must be approached with patience, gentle persuasion and, when necessary, firmness. He should be encouraged to become involved in the everyday activities of the unit. However, he is unlikely to apply himself to any particular activity, including physical exercise, for very long.

PARANOID STATES

Psychiatric illness in certain elderly people manifests itself as delusional beliefs of a persecutory nature. Paranoid delusions can occur in a number of conditions including acute confusional states, depression, dementia, hypothyroidism and drug intoxication. Sensory deprivation, especially deafness and, to a lesser extent, blindness, predispose to paranoia. All patients who are deaf should be encouraged to wear a hearing aid otherwise social isolation is likely to occur as a consequence of the severe communication problems. The strange environment of a hospital may also precipitate paranoia and many elderly people feel very threatened by modern technological medicine.

Apart from being found in the conditions and situations mentioned already, paranoia may also be due to paraphrenia. This mental disorder is found typically in elderly partially deaf females without a previous history of serious psychiatric illness. They are often rather eccentric and isolated. The individual becomes suspicious about the people around her and as the illness progresses she may hear hallucinatory voices. Nothing is achieved by challenging the patient about her delusions and she imagines she is being spied upon. The symptoms usually respond readily to tranquillisers. Sometimes paranoid delusions are a manifestation of a frank schizophrenic illness but usually these patients have a long history of schizophrenia. It is rare for a patient to develop a schizophrenic illness for the first time in old age.

CONFUSION

Acute confusion is a common mode of presentation of illness in the older patient. It is essential to assess the patient very thoroughly for an underlying illness. Acute confusion, for instance, can be the presenting feature of a number of life-threatening conditions such as myocardial infarction, pneumonia, pulmonary embolism and gastro-intestinal bleeding. Drugs are a common cause of acute confusion in the elderly. As emphasised earlier, older patients cannot adapt to change as readily as younger patients and a change of environment in itself can produce confusion. The patient is disoriented, thought processes and memory are impaired and the level of alertness may fluctuate. Illusions, hallucinations and delusions are present. Illusions or false perceptions about the environment are particularly likely to occur in a dimly lit environment. Delusions are usually paranoid and the patient may become quite aggressive.

Acute confusion is caused by the effect of the precipitating illness on the brain. This may be brought about by factors such as toxins, impaired cerebral metabolism, hypoxia, electrolyte imbalance or dehydration. The confusion will begin to resolve if the underlying physical condition responds to appropriate therapy.

Confident and caring staff will reassure the patient and hasten the return to normality. However, if the staff are unsure, rejecting and negative in their approach, the chances of recovery are impeded. Sedation should be used judiciously. The acute confusional state usually ends fairly quickly with either recovery or with the death of the patient. Only very rarely does it develop into a chronic dementing process.

SENILE DEMENTIA

Senile dementia is defined as the global impairment of higher cortical function. The ability to cope with the performance of daily activities is impaired but consciousness is not. Microscopic changes are found in the neurons of the cerebral cortex. Alzheimer (1907) described abnormal tangles of small filaments in these cells, known as neurofibrillary tangles. Apart from the tangles, there are collections of degenerating nerve endings known as neuritic plaques. The most notable biochemical change which has been observed in the brain tissue of dementing patients is the low level of acetyl transferase, the enzyme which forms the neurotransmitter substance acetylcholine. The disease is primarily a condition of the elderly, but it also occurs in younger adults (presenile dementia).

One of the earliest features of the condition is a deterioration of memory for recent events and an inability to plan ahead. Further intellectual decline leads to frank confusion, language disturbances, apraxia, a tendency to wander, agitation and difficulty in performing the activities of daily living. The patient becomes incontinent and increasingly immobile. The rate of decline varies from individual to individual and ranges from months to years. As the disease progresses, the patient loses insight. In a sense this is fortunate and they need considerable support.

Physiotherapy may help to preserve the patient's declining mobility as the disease progresses. Therapy should be carried out in a quiet atmosphere. Instructions given to the patient should be clear and simple and the therapist should stand where she can be seen easily. The patient should be reassured when necessary and conflict should be avoided. The use of calendars and clocks and other appropriate cues may be of considerable benefit and occupational therapists should be able to help in this 'reality orientation'. Even the most debilitated older patient retains some ability to learn new information. Although conditioned responses may be acquired more slowly in the aged, the older patient can learn new verbal material, new motor skills and new problem-solving strategies. Those patients who cannot perform a learned motor movement although their strength is intact (apraxia) may also benefit from physiotherapy. The difficulty might lie in one part of a complex movement and this may be identified if the movement is broken down into its different components. A strategy can then be devised that might help the patient and relatives to overcome the difficulty. Patients with apraxia may be unable to learn new skills. It might not be possible, for instance, to treat a patient with diminished mobility how to use a walking aid. It would of course be hazardous to give an aid to a patient who cannot use it properly. More can be achieved by personal interest, involvement and stimulation in such patients than can be achieved by medication. The familiar should be used to maintain the patient's contact with reality, and if institutional care is necessary, it is helpful to have some familiar objects such as photographs, ornaments, items of small clothing or small furnishings available for the person to see or use in an environment that is otherwise totally strange. The patient's cat, for instance, may be a useful reminder of home and in some centres, pets are a welcome addition to the ward. Considerable research is currently taking place, but as yet there is no 'cure' for the condition.

Each case should be investigated appropriately, as treatable conditions such as subdural haematoma, brain tumour, metabolic or nutritional abnormalities should be excluded. Normal pressure hydrocephalus is a syndrome that consists of progressive intellectual decline, rigidity and akinesia, urinary incontinence and gait disturbance. Marked enlargement of the cerebral ventricles is shown on a CT scan. The insertion of a shunt by a neurosurgeon may lead to improvement. It has particular relevance to the physiotherapist as those patients with gait disturbance and a mild degree of mental disturbance have the best outlook after surgery. The condition should always be borne in mind.

Cerebrovascular disease can also lead to dementia by causing multiple infarcts throughout the brain, so-called multi-infarct dementia. The patients are usually hypertensive, they have a short-stepped gait and increased tone of spastic quality. There is usually other evidence of cerebrovascular and cardiovascular disease.

Physiotherapy

The physiotherapist is most likely to be asked to assess a patient with early Alzheimer-type disease in order to help the team to define which functional disabilities are due to loss of cognitive powers and which are due to other specific physical causes. During the later stages of the illness, the therapist may be involved in treating physical complications and advising relatives and nurses on appropriate care. Patients with advanced multi-infarct dementia tend to suffer from contractures, so it is important to make every effort to maintain as full a range of movement at all joints as is possible. However, in some patients, it is virtually impossible to avoid some degree of contracture. Pain often accompanies spasm and it may be thought by the patient that the physiotherapist is the cause of the pain. Hare (1986) has commented upon the importance of careful handling of such patients and of providing appropriate support for injured and painful limbs.

REALITY ORIENTATION

The procedure of reality orientation, described by Folsom (1968), Drummond, Kirckhoff and Scarbrough (1978) and Holden and

Woods (1982) aims to reintroduce a confused person to the environment by continuous, repetitive orientation stimuli. It consists of two
components: basic 24-hour orientation and classroom orientation.
Twenty-four hour reality orientation consists of constant reminders
given to the confused person to relate them to time, place and person
by verbal and visual stimuli, such as signs, clocks, calendars, direc-
tional arrows and personal belongings. Time is allowed for patients
to respond to stimuli and appropriate answers are rewarded with
praise. Classroom orientation supplements the 24-hour treatment
with short, intensive periods for small groups of selected patients.
Sessions are best held in special accommodation that is bright, and
attractively equipped, again with interesting and stimulating material
in the room. Classes may be taken at basic and progressive levels
(Hare 1986).

The value of reality orientation has only been examined critically
relatively recently. Early studies relied on subjective impressions.
Harris and Ivory (1976), Woods (1979) and Hanley, McGuire and
Boyd (1981), using standard scales and inventories, demonstrated
that classroom reality-orientation produced some improvement in
verbal orientation, but no improvement in behaviour, unlike Barnes'
(1974) earlier study, which did find qualitative improvement.
Hanley *et al.* (1981) questioned the effort required to train a team
leader in relation to the degree of improvement attained by the
patient. They found that 24-hour reality orientation improved ward
orientation and behaviour and these effects overshadowed the minor
improvements in verbal orientation produced by classroom orientation. Brooks, Degun and Mather (1975) demonstrated that the least
disoriented, more intellectually and socially oriented patients
obtained most benefit from such treatment. Whether the improvements are due to the treatment programme, or to the increased attention of staff is disputed. The technique has been shown to help the
elderly in a residential home in terms of orientation but not in terms
of the activities of daily living (Zepelin, Wolfe and Kleinplatz 1977).

Sutcliffe (1983) comments that the two forms of reality orientation both have a considerable contribution to make to the life of a
long-stay geriatric ward. Such a treatment regime demands that staff
give maximum care to patients, which is to be welcomed and should
be considered the right of the patient. The implication of this
approach to care is that information about the locality of the ward,
the hospital, the day, the date and the time is conspicuously posted
in the ward area. Patient areas should be signposted: the doors
leading to the toilet areas, the dayrooms and the bedrooms should

be labelled in upper and lower case letters. Beds and lockers should be identified individually with large nameplates and perhaps specially designed boards. As well as providing all these visual cues, the staff must consciously try to involve the patient in using these reminders. If someone asks the time, staff members can first ask him if he sees the clock so that, in fact, the patient is afforded the opportunity to tell the staff member the time. During dressing, the staff member can ask if they have noticed the weather outdoors, if it is raining, if the sun is shining, if the wind is blowing and so on and if such weather is appropriate for the time of the year.

A reality-orientation board (notice board) should be in a prominent position in the ward and rest areas and should display the date, comments on the weather and points of interest; information is changed daily. The format is similar to that found in many primary or national schools and playgroups.

Classroom orientation may be conducted in small groups (three to five patients), though this may have to be adapted if a patient has speech, visual or hearing disabilities. The session might begin with a general introduction of all members of the group, who would then in turn read the information on the orientation board. The daily news, happenings on the ward and the menu for lunch or dinner could then be discussed. Simple games may also be played during the session, which could involve identification of objects and communication between members of the group. The session should end with a review of names and of the information on the orientation board.

PSYCHOGERIATRIC SERVICE

In recent years, an increasing number of psychiatrists have responded to the challenge of mental illness in the elderly in the UK. In some areas, they have developed a comprehensive service for these patients. Although many elderly patients with mental disability will be looked after by the primary health-care team in the community, the support of an efficient psychogeriatric service has proven itself to be of great value. The presence of such a service creates a higher degree of awareness of the problem and more patients with remediable illness are detected early (Godber 1983). Successful departments have both community and hospital facilities and they work closely with the geriatric department and other specialist services involved in caring for the elderly. In certain areas, the psychiatrist and geriatrician operate joint assessment wards and clinics where the patients' mental and physical problems can be fully evaluated.

The techniques of physiotherapy are no different for psycho-geriatric patients than for any other elderly patient. However, the pace is often slower and the skill is in adapting common practice to the states of mental stress exhibited by the patients. The physio-therapist may be involved in treating patients at home, in a day hospital or in a hospital or other institution. The aim is to keep the patient in his own environment for as long as possible.

Patients with advanced dementia begin to develop physical problems. Sometimes these problems are related to medication, for example extrapyramidal signs secondary to phenothiazine therapy, but often they are an integral part of the disease process. Sometimes long-stay care in an institution becomes inevitable either because of increasing disability or the presence of a level of mental impairment that cannot be coped with in the community. The primary objective of physiotherapy in this situation is to maintain mobility and to co-operate with other members of the team in making the environment as homely as possible for the patients. A movement group may be used to considerable advantage. All members of staff should be encouraged to assist in mobilising the patients. The physiotherapist should work in close co-operation with the occupational therapist, providing the patients with the opportunity to undertake activities that are as lively and purposeful as possible. Working together like this, they will maintain the patients' optimal independence in carry-ing out the activities of daily living.

REFERENCES

Alzheimer, A. (1907) 'Ueber eine Eigencotige Enarankung der Hirnrinde.' *Col. Nervenheilk Psychiat. 18*, 177

Barnes, J. (1974) 'Effects of reality orientation classroom on memory loss, confusion and disorientation in geriatric patients.' *Gerontologist, 14*, 138–42

Bergmann, K. (1979) 'Neurosis and personality disorders in old age.' In A. Isaacs and F. Post (eds), *Geriatric Psychiatry*, Wiley, Chichester

Brooks, P., Degun, G. and Mather, M. (1975) 'Reality orientation, a therapy for psychogeriatric patients. A controlled study.' *Brit. J. Psychol. 127*, 42–5

Coakley, D. and Woodford-Williams, P. (1979) 'Effects of burglary and vandalism in the homes of old people.' *Lancet, ii*, 1066–7

Droller, H. (1964) 'Some aspects of alcoholism in the elderly.' *Lancet, ii*, 137–9

Drummond, L., Kirckhoff, L. and Scarbrough, D.R. (1978) 'A practical guide to reality orientation: a treatment approach for confusion and disorientation.' *Gerontologist, 18*, 568–73

Folsom, J.C. (1968) 'Reality orientation for the elderly mental patient.' *J. Geriat. Psychiatry, 1*, 291–306

Godber, C. (1983) 'Depression in Old Age.' *Brit. Med. J. [Clin. Res.] 287*, 758

Hanley, I.G., McGuire, R.J. and Boyd, W.D. (1981) 'Reality orientation and dementia: a controlled trial of two approaches.' *Brit. J. Psychiatry, 183*, 10–14

Hare, M. (1986) *Physiotherapy in psychiatry.* Heinemann, London

Harris, C.S. and Ivory, P.B.C.B. (1976) 'An outcome evaluation of reality orientation therapy with geriatric patients in a state mental hospital.' *Gerontologist, 16*, 496–503

Holden, U. and Woods, R. (1982) *Reality orientation.* Churchill Livingstone, Edinburgh

Kay, D. and Beamish, P. (1964) 'Old age mental disorders in Newcastle-upon-Tyne.' *Brit. J. Psychiatry, 110*, 146

Pitt, B. (1982) *Psychogeriatrics.* Churchill Livingstone, Edinburgh

Post, F. (1978) 'Psychiatric disorders.' In J.C. Brocklehurst (ed), *Textbook of geriatric medicine and gerontology*, Churchill Livingstone, Edinburgh

Sutcliffe, B.J. (1983) 'Improving quality of life in psychogeriatric units.' In M.J. Denham (ed), *Care of the long stay elderly patient*, Croom Helm, London

Woods, R.T. (1979) 'Reality orientation and staff attention: a controlled study.' *Brit. J. Psychiatry, 134*, 502–7

Zepelin, H., Wolfe, C.S. and Kleinplatz, F. (1977) 'Evaluation of a year long reality orientation program.' *J. Gerontol., 36*, 70–7

11

Music, Leisure and Exercise

References to music and medicine are common in Greek and Latin literature (Henson 1977). Early writers were concerned with the therapeutic effects of music: Plumy in 1513 reported that Cato had preserved an incantation for the cure of sprains and Varo another for gout. Aureliaus in 1529 mentioned the use of music in the general treatment of insanity and sciatica. In 1632 Burton, in his reference to music, presented the art as a remedy for morbid states of mind, 'Many men are melancholy by hearing music but it is a pleasing melancholy that it causeth, and therefore to such as are discontent, in woe, fear, sorrow or dejected it is a most pleasing remedy. It expels cares, alters their grieved minds and easeth in an instant.' However, despite these early writings, it was not until after World War II, with the occurrence of a great number of cases of 'shell shock', that new approaches to psychiatric medicine became necessary and music therapy received great emphasis.

Over the past couple of decades, the trend in medical care has been towards the total-care approach (Bright 1972). However, because of the specialisation of different aspects of treatment, it is sometimes difficult to achieve such a unified approach. Music can enter into many aspects of care and so act as a cohesive force binding together a diversity of treatments. In most musical activities, the patient has some degree of choice in what is done — the songs to be sung and the music to be played. Physiotherapy is often difficult for a patient and sometimes it is a painful experience. These factors, added to those imposed by advancing age and disability, may add up to an unbearable sense of restraint and frustration. Music provides each individual with the chance to express himself as a person.

Isolation is a common phenomenon among the ageing population and for many, it is the cause of grave loneliness and depression.

Isolation produces severe guilt feelings in certain people, with a resultant depressive psychosis (Sloane 1970). In other cases, the depressed person adopts a 'sick role' thereby reducing and modifying what is expected of him in life and increasing the amount of attention he will receive. There are several causes of isolation and possible consequent loneliness: bereavement, separation from children, retirement, with the consequent loss of a sense of achievement and usefulness, and physical disabilities. Johnson (1960) states that loneliness may well be called the greatest problem of the aged. Music may evoke associations with a happier past. Colours, scents and sounds will all have the power to take the patient back in time and to relive the past. Sometimes the memories will be unpleasant, but more often, pleasant. There are frequently pleasant memories associated with memories of love and courtship. Songs associated with both World Wars may have happy memories, reminding the patient of friends and the recollection of being needed by the community. Music therapy should be used to encourage discussion, relating one patient's memories to those of others in the group. At a music conference in Canada, one delegate commented that music could be an unblocker of emotions; it can give comfort non-verbally, whilst motivating the weary to live.

McGreal (1984) carried out a small pilot study using groups of elderly patients attending a day hospital; their mean age was 72. The two groups were treated over a three-week period, one group exercising to music and a second group exercising without music. Both classes consisted of the same twelve simple activities, which were selected with the aim of helping patients to cope better with activities of daily living and to achieve mobility of joints. McGreal concluded from the study that music does have a stimulating effect on movement and that it should be considered as part of the rehabilitation programme for the elderly.

LEISURE AND EXERCISE

The traditional pattern of hospital care is often poorly suited to the elderly person. The danger of institutionalisation is a very real one. The very structure of a hospital, with its hierarchy still very evident in many cases, positively encourages a docile, co-operative, submissive patient, in whom motivation and initiative are neither sought nor actively encouraged.

One of the most pronounced changes that accompanies old age is loss of mobility. Elderly people often avoid certain activities, such as climbing stairs, walking, etc., because of instability. We live in an age of advanced technology in which the many labour-saving devices that are available limit the activity an elderly person needs to do. It is not uncommon to hear an old person being told to slow down, or to take it easy, advice meant in the best sense, but encouraging inactivity of body and mind. Leisure is a valuable part of life, and elderly people have an opportunity to avail themselves of it. Leisure time should provide stimulation, challenge and enjoyment for the elderly person and there are therefore many advantages to be gained from a positive approach. Some people will be fortunate to remain fit enough to continue such activities as riding, golf, swimming, etc. Various limitations will lead others to less-active pursuits like bowling, cards, billiards and chess. Grandchildren often take up an interest from their grandparents, for example, in activities such as photography or collecting things such as stamps, matchboxes, prints, china, etc. Some elderly people pick up a paintbrush for the first time in their lives. The art therapist plays an increasingly important role both in rehabilitation and in continuing care environments (see Fig. 11.1). Many old people enjoy gardening and there are means of reducing some of the hard labour involved through a variety of garden tools on the market. The use of raised flower beds, greenhouses and indoor gardens can foster much enthusiasm and happiness. Swimming is an ideal activity for the older age group as it combines both leisure and therapy. Older people are more likely to swim if there are age-banded sessions for the elderly. They tend not to like to swim in sessions available to the general public because of the noise and the fear of being jostled and hampered by younger users of the pool (MacHeath 1984). Other common activities in which the elderly seek pleasure are fishing, reading, walking, driving for pleasure, visiting friends and relatives and attending clubs and organisations. This is not an over-demanding group of activities, yet in most, a physical ability is a requirement.

Exercise is not just for the young, though there will be inevitable limitations on the elderly. It has been pointed out that if all elderly people with 'abnormalities' in their electrocardiographs were prohibited from exercising, few senior citizens would move, although there is no categorical information of the risks involved. Advancing age is accompanied by loss of strength and reduced speed of movement. Observation has shown that the elderly use a restricted range of movement as their daily activities do not require the maximum range of movement. Bone loss is associated with ageing and osteoporotic bone is weaker than normal bone (See Chapter 6). Reddan (1981) states that although structural and functional changes associated with age result in a decline in respiratory function, the degree and rate of loss is variable and dependent upon the overall health of the individual. Many young people show the same structural and functional changes.

How then might a safe programme of activity be planned for a healthy, elderly population ? Cowan (1974) postulated that although old age is a part of normal, human development, our culture so distorts this phenomenon that most people are afraid to face up to it. In a survey of a particular district health authority in England, MacHeath (1984) found that, in many instances, the current generation of elderly people, both men and women, have a greater level of participation in leisure activities than younger generations, with only a modest decline in the over-80s group. In her study, those aged over 80 compared favourably with the staff under 40 years old who were caring for them at clubs for the elderly! There are those who seem to be little affected by their age and can continue with normal habits and activities; while at the other end of the spectrum, there are those who are hindered by multiple pathology. In this latter group, there is a need for a minimum level of daily exercise to prevent problems associated with immobility (Saltin *et al.* 1968).

Before embarking on a programme of exercise, the older, more mobile person needs to be assessed in order to identify those who may be at risk. Standard tests need to be modified for the elderly. For instance, many do not cope well with a treadmill and they may be quite unable to walk normally on a moving surface. In the literature, it has been shown clearly in terms of energy expenditure that the values associated with outdoor circuits are closely similar to those associated with walking on a treadmill (Haisman, Winsmann and Goldman 1972). The velocity of gait should fall within the range 2 kmhr^{-1} to 5 kmhr^{-1}, as Margaria (1976) has shown that energy requirement is independent of speed over this range, at about 0.5 kCal kg^{-1} km^{-1}. A bicycle ergometer, though easier for the subject to balance on, also suffers limitations if a patient suffers leg pain or weakness, or if his co-ordination is impaired. The simplest form of testing is probably a modified Harvard Step Test. Morse (1981) used a step height of 10.2–30.5 cm (4–12 inches), provoking a heart rate of 75% of a predicted maximum heart rate (at 24–30 steps per minute). A handhold is permitted for support and security.

In creating an exercise programme, the following factors must be taken into account:

1. Age and ability level;
2. The interests of those involved;
3. Objectives need to be defined;
4. The social need of those involved;
5. Competitiveness.

The ability level is of greater importance than age when reviewing the possibility of taking a number of elderly people together. It is counter-productive when a randomly selected group of non-specific exercises are demonstrated to a non-motivated group of patients by an equally unenthusiastic physiotherapist. The effect is total boredom for all concerned and any therapeutic value achieved is accomplished by chance. The aim of activity should be to increase social contact. Although individual exercises play an important part in rehabilitation, there has to be a place for group activity. Husbands or wives and close friends ought to be encouraged to attend. The activities that are selected for group activity in the elderly should minimise negative, competitive feelings and differences among personalities involved. This does not mean that all competition should be avoided, but it should be evolved by the participants not created or demanded by the physiotherapist. Participants should be advised to exercise within their own comfortable limits and not push themselves to be seen to be doing better than a neighbour.

Morse (1981) described what he termed a 'fitness trail'. Exercise is conducted on three days a week for twelve weeks, each session lasting for about one hour. Sessions begin with a warm-up for ten to fifteen minutes including chair exercises and stretching and some general announcements of interest to the group. The participants then divide into groups. The trail is divided into quarter-mile lengths, with exercise stations at the intervals. At each interval, exercises that aim at strength, flexibility and co-ordination are completed. Later, the intervals between the exercise stations are increased. The fitness trail is designed for outdoor activity which, in some countries, because of the vagaries of the weather, could present problems. However, modification for indoor use would not be impossible.

What are the benefits of exercise in the elderly? Chapman, de Vries and Sweezey (1972) have shown that exercise can produce increases in strength in the elderly that are similar in magnitude to those that would be expected in younger subjects. Sidney (1981)

177

demonstrated that appropriate programmes of activity over an eight-week period can bring about cardiovascular adaptations in the elderly that are similar to adaptations brought about in both young and middle-aged adults. The difficulty is to discover the most suitable combination of intensity, frequency and duration that will bring about an optimal response. Joints are most flexible in the middle 20s and flexibility decreases with age (Munns 1981). Most of the stiffness in a joint in the elderly is in the soft tissues — muscle, tendons and joint capsule. Exercises designed to act on these areas of the body could potentially increase range of movement in the elderly by reducing stiffness (Chapman *et al.* 1972). Munns (1981) significantly increased range of movement using a programme of exercise and dance; the participants met three times a week for twelve weeks. The programme of activity must be relevant and of interest, because as the range of movement improves, not only will subjects find an increase in general comfort, but also an increase in the number of activities in which they can take part. A suggested programme of activity is shown in Appendix II, p. 215.

Certain investigators have concluded that physical training in individuals over the age of 40 is only moderately effective and claim that past the age of 60, there is no observable effect achieved (Hollman 1964). Others have shown that a significant improvement is achieved in the capacity for physical work with regulated exercise programmes (Skinner 1970). Perkins and Kaiser (1961) in a classic weight-resisted exercise programme conjectured that it would be wise to consider preventive resisted exercises for the aged populations of nursing homes as a means of retraining functional ability and reducing the need for care. de Vries (1970) concluded that the potential of training elderly men is probably greater than had been suspected and does not depend upon having trained in youth.

Patterson (1986), in a study of the effects of regular exercise classes on a group of patients in long-term residential care in Ireland, found a significant increase in function, increased motivation and socialisation among patients. The activities used in this study are shown in Appendix III p. 217. It is sometimes claimed that there is not time to organise exercise classes for elderly patients. However, Patterson has demonstrated that the time taken to organise and give a class can reduce the need for individual therapy and decrease potential cases of apathetic and immobile patients. She found that patients responded well and showed an increase in functional mobility apart from enjoying the social element of the sessions.

Physical exercise increases body temperature and fluid loss becomes more pronounced through sweating and respiration. In the elderly, the diminished sensitivity of the thermostatic mechanism results in higher temperatures; cooling is less efficient because its onset is delayed and sweating surfaces are reduced. In overheated rooms therefore, exercise programmes may become hazardous for the elderly person (Hunt 1983). While sweating as a result of heating and exercise may be less in the elderly, thirst is also lessened and fluid intake may be insufficient to overcome increases in ventilatory losses. It is important therefore that aged persons have frequent rest periods in their rehabilitation activities to allow for cooling and fluid intake. Elderly patients should always have fluid readily available to them during their exercise class. Best results are achieved from exercise classes if they take place during the morning (Hunt 1980).

The work of Patterson concurs with that of Connolly (1986) who investigated the effects of physiotherapy on the mobility of the elderly in long-term care. In her study, she demonstrated a significant improvement in mobility in patients who were treated daily compared to those who were treated twice a week or not at all.

Residents in long-term care suffer from the effects of institutionalisation — dependency, attention-seeking behaviour and abnormal possessiveness (Townsend 1962). As admissions are often as a result of social problems, many patients are quite mobile on admission. A few months after admission, it is frequently noted that there is a decrease in mobility and function. Visitors may attend infrequently and so most communication is with staff members. Interaction with and attention from staff tends to be greatest among dependent residents. Such dependence may arise from attention-seeking behaviour. If patients notice other residents being attended to more than themselves, they may be tempted to become dependent. Regular activity can help alleviate the effects of institutionalisation and Skeist (1980) suggested that there is a greater sense of commitment when working daily as opposed to working twice weekly.

REFERENCES

Bright, R. (1972) *Music in geriatric care*. Angus and Robertson, Glasgow
Chapman, E.A., de Vries, H.A. and Sweezey, R. (1972) 'Joint stiffness: effects of exercise on young and old men.' *J. Gerontol. 27*, 218–24
Connolly, C.S. (1986) 'Evaluation of physiotherapy among elderly residents in extended care', Project submitted, University of Dublin

179

Cowan, N.R. (1974) 'Preventive aspects of geriatrics.' In W.F. Anderson (ed), *Geriatric medicine*, Academic Press, London

de Vries, H.A. (1970) 'Physiological effects of an exercise programme upon men aged 52–88 years.' *J. Gerontol.*, *25*, 325–31

Haisman, M.F., Winsmann, F.R. and Goldman, R.F. (1972) 'Energy cost of pushing loaded handcarts.' *J. Appl. Physiol.*, *32*(3), 181–6

Henson, C.M. (1977) *Music and the brain: studies in the neurology of music*. William Heinemann Medical Books, London

Hollman, W. (1964) 'Changes in the capacity for maximal and continuous effort in relation to age.' In E. Johl and E. Simon (eds), *Environmental research in sports and physical education*, Charles C. Thomas, Springfield, Illinois

Hunt, T.M. (1983) 'Practical considerations in the rehabilitation of the aged.' *J. Am. Ger. Soc. 28*, 2

Johnson, E. (1960) 'Society provisions for the aged in Australian society.' *Australian J. of Ger.*, *60*, 45–53

McGreal, A. (1984) 'Music in physiotherapy — an approach in the rehabilitation of the elderly', Project submitted, University of Dublin

MacHeath, J.A. (1984) *Activity, health and fitness in old age*. Croom Helm, London

Margaria, R. (1976) *Biomechanics and analysis of muscular exercise*. Clarendon Press, Oxford

Morse, C.E. (1981) 'Physical activity programming for the aged,' In E. Smith and R. Serfass (eds), *Exercise and ageing*, Enslow Publishers, New Jersey

Munns, K. (1981) 'Effects of exercise in the range of joint motion in elderly patients.' In E. Smith and R. Serfass (eds), *Exercise and ageing*, Enslow Publishers, New Jersey

Patterson, J. (1986) 'An evaluation of the need of the long-stay elderly patient for an organised exercise class', Project submitted, University of Dublin

Perkins, L.C. and Kaiser, H.L. (1961) 'Results of short term isotonic and isometric exercise programmes in persons over 60 years.' *Phys. Ther. Rev.*, *41*, 633–9

Reddan, W.G. (1981) 'Respiratory system and ageing.' In E. Smith and R. Serfass (eds), *Exercise and ageing*, Enslow Publishers, New Jersey

Saltin, B., Blomquist, G., Michell, J.H., Johnson, R.L., Wildenthal, K. and Chapman, C.B. (1968) 'Response to exercise after bed rest and after training.' *Circul. Suppl.*, *7*, 1

Sidney, K.H. (1981) 'Cardiovascular benefits of physical activity in the aged.' In E. Smith and R. Serfass (eds), *Exercise and ageing*, Enslow Publishers, New Jersey

Skeist, M. (1980) 'Role of physical therapists in a physical activity programme in nursing homes: a survey.' *J. Am. Ger. Soc.*, *27*, 3

Skinner, J. (1970) 'The cardiovascular system with ageing and exercise'. In D. Brunner and E. Jokl (eds), *Medicine in sport*, *vol.4*, *Physical activity and ageing*, University Press, Baltimore

Sloane, F.D. (1970) 'The mentally afflicted older person.' *J. of Geriat.*, *11*, 73–82

Townsend, P. (1962) *The last refuge*. Routledge and Keegan Paul, London

12

Medication and Physiotherapy

Drugs are more likely to cause side effects in older rather than in younger patients. One might expect, then, that drugs would be used very sparingly in the older age group. In fact, the opposite is true and it is not uncommon to see an old person on several different medications. Some drugs have side effects that lead to increased muscular rigidity and/or immobility. Others can cause problems such as drowsiness, incontinence, unsteadiness, falls and confusion. Drug treatment can therefore lead to disability resulting in the need for physiotherapy or, in other instances, it can greatly impede the patient's ability to co-operate with the physiotherapist. It is therefore important that the physiotherapist should have an appreciation of how drugs are handled by the elderly and also of the pitfalls in therapeutics in this age group.

The way a drug is dealt with by the body is usually described under four headings: absorption, distribution, metabolism and excretion. The physiological changes of ageing affect all four processes.

ABSORPTION

Most drugs taken by mouth are absorbed by passive diffusion into the blood stream. The process of absorption can be slowed by using enteric-coated or sustained-release formulations. Many physiological factors influence drug absorption such as the pH of the gastrointestinal tract, the rate of gastric emptying, intestinal motility and the absorptive surface of the small intestine. Although age changes may affect all of these functions, it is thought that drug absorption is not appreciably altered in old age (Crooks, O'Malley and Stevenson 1976). Thus, even though age changes may reduce the absorptive surface of the small intestine, this is unlikely to be significant as the remaining absorptive area is still about the size of two full-sized tennis courts! (MacDonald and MacDonald 1982.)

DISTRIBUTION

Drugs are transported in the circulation largely bound to plasma proteins. These proteins have several sites capable of forming reversible bonds with drug molecules of different shape. Some drugs may compete for the same binding sites and this will have obvious practical implications for therapy, particularly in the elderly, where many drugs are often used in the same patient. Serum-protein levels drop with age and this decline may be aggravated by chronic disease and immobility. This change means that there are higher levels of unbound drug in the circulation and as it is the unbound 'free' form that is metabolically active, there can be important therapeutic implications. For example, the sedative diazepam is over 97 per cent bound to protein in the circulation so that a drop of a few per cent in protein-binding would increase the blood levels of the active fraction by approximately 100 per cent. One must therefore be cautious in treating elderly patients with highly bound protein drugs such as diazepam. Body fat increases with age and the amount of lean body mass diminishes. Because of this, drugs such as digoxin, which are highly bound to tissue proteins will have smaller distribution volumes and elevated serum levels in the elderly. Fat-soluble drugs on the other hand will have a larger distribution volume because there is more fatty tissue. Most drugs are fat soluble and because of the extra storage area, their effect may be prolonged in the elderly. In particular, many hypnotics and sedatives are fat soluble.

METABOLISM

Drugs can be divided into two basic groups — fat-soluble and water-soluble. Water-soluble drugs are excreted unchanged by the kidney and for these, renal function is critical. Fat-soluble drugs are reabsorbed by the kidney nephrons and so they must be metabolised to water-soluble compounds before they can be excreted by the kidneys. The liver plays a central role in their metabolism and impaired hepatic function in the elderly is likely to be a factor in the increased incidence of drug toxicity in this age group. For instance, the metabolism of the sedative chlordiazepoxide is slower in older people.

EXCRETION

Most drugs are excreted by the kidney. Renal blood flow and glomerular filtration at the age of 75 are about 50 per cent of the level in younger adults. Particular care must be exercised when using drugs with a low safety margin. Slight changes in the blood levels of these drugs can lead to serious toxicity. For instance, the antibiotics penicillin and aminoglycoside are both excreted by the kidneys. The first drug has a wide safety margin so that problems are unlikely to arise unless renal function is severely reduced. In contrast, mild renal impairment can lead to serious problems such as ototoxicity if aminoglycosides are administered without care, as they have a very narrow safety margin.

INCREASED ORGAN SENSITIVITY

Apart from the differences in the way the body deals with drugs between different age groups, there is also evidence that ageing tissues may be more sensitive to the effects of nitrazepam, a commonly used hypnotic, as well as to the phenothiazines.

PERIOD OF ACTION

Some drugs are cleared quickly from the body and this is an advantage when using drugs such as sedatives and hypnotics. For instance, the hypnotic chlormethiazole is quickly cleared from the blood stream. However, nitrazepam, is cleared much more slowly and may cause problems such as over-sedation, unsteadiness and confusion on the day following its administration.

MEDICATION AND PHYSIOTHERAPY

It is vital that the physiotherapist should know which drugs the patient is taking. For instance, the patient may be on drugs that improve mobility such as levodopa and checks should be made that they are actually being taken. Poor response is often related to poor compliance with the drug regime. It is useful to actually see the bottles, as a patient may be confused about the medication. One should also be sure that the patient has the manual dexterity to be able to open the drug packs or bottles.

Drugs can impede a patient's rehabilitation in several ways. For example, postural hypotension will make the patient unsteady and inclined to fall, thus decreasing confidence. Many drugs can cause postural hypotension, including tricyclic antidepressants, antihypertensive agents, diuretics, levodopa and phenothiazines. Fatigue is a common complaint of patients on diuretics and beta-blocking drugs. Some antihypertensive drugs such as methyldopa and reserpine also cause fatigue and of course it is common with sedatives and antidepressants. Some drugs such as benztropine, bromocriptine, amantadine, cimetidine, indomethacin, levodopa, methyldopa and reserpine can cause frank depression. Depressed patients will not respond optimally to physiotherapy. There are also many drugs that can cause confusional reactions, including commonly used drugs such as digoxin and aminophylline. Incontinence may be precipitated by diuretics as well as by drugs that impair mobility. Drug-induced parkinsonism is commonly seen in old people. Phenothiazines, haloperidol and metachlopramide are drugs that may produce extrapyramidal side effects. If antipsychotic agents are prescribed, a close watch should be kept for these side effects. The extrapyramidal signs do not respond to levodopa, but significant improvement may be seen with anticholinergic drugs. Involuntary movements of the mouth and jaw (tardive dyskinesia) are other unpleasant side effects of these drugs.

VERTIGO AND DIZZINESS

Recent studies have shown that drugs can be a major cause of dizziness in the elderly (Gomolin and Chapron 1983; Blumenthal and Davie 1980). Some drugs such as gentamycin, amikacin, fenoprofen, ibuproven, indomethacin and naproxen may cause vestibular damage. Ataxia is particularly prevalent with benzodiazepines and anticonvulsants.

Many other drugs may cause disability that might bring a patient to the physiotherapist. An alert and vigilant therapist may be the first person to connect the disability with the patient's medication.

REFERENCES

Blumenthal, M.D. and Davie, J.W. (1980) 'Dizziness and falling in elderly psychiatric out-patients.' *Am. J. Psychiat.*, *137*(2), 203–6

Crooks, J., O'Malley, K. and Stevenson, I.H. (1976) 'Pharmacokinetics in the elderly.' *Clin. Pharmacokinet.*, *1*(4), 280–96

Gomolin, I.H. and Chapron, D.J. (1983) 'Rational drug therapy for the aged.' *Compr. Ther.*, *9*(7), 17–30

MacDonald, R.A. and MacDonald, B.E. (1982) 'Alcoholism in residency program candidates.' *J. Med. Educ. 57*(9), 692–5

13

Care of the Dying

In this century, there has been a dramatic change in the age at which people die. This is largely due to improved social conditions and, to a lesser extent, to advances in medical treatment. This movement of the time of death from the young to the old has had a major effect on our society. Very few physiotherapy students witness a death before beginning their training. This would not have been the case earlier in the century. The modern lack of contact with the realities of birth, life and death makes it more difficult for health professionals to cope with the problems of dying patients.

Physiotherapists do not particularly associate themselves with the care of the dying, yet they form an important part of the team. Most terminally ill patients have been treated by several different team members for some time before the final phase of their illness. It is essential therefore that they should not feel deserted at this critical and often frightening stage by those workers with whom they have built up a relationship during therapy (Charleton and Coles 1982). Care of the dying is an area which is different to 'normal' work. There is, for example, a tendency to be too eager, to take over all aspects of care, leaving both patient and relatives with little to do and feeling excluded and useless. In the area of terminal care, it is not only the patient who receives care, but also the relatives and friends who visit; they will all be facing a crisis in their lives. The fact that a patient is dying should not alter his rights. The rights of the dying patient are no different from those of other patients, except that the dying might have a greater claim on our attention. We owe it to the patient to respect his rights. The dying patient may be anxious to talk to someone about personal, financial, moral and spiritual problems. The caring physiotherapist, who may spend much time on a one-to-one basis with a patient, may be the person with whom the dying patient may talk and she has the obligation to respect the patient's confidences. She should refrain from imposing personal views. Sympathetic listening and encouragement will help the patient to find his own answers, or to seek appropriate help and advice from others.

The second right is the right to treatment (or to refuse it). Interpreted too narrowly, it would oblige the physiotherapist to assist in the maintenance of life for as long as possible, with scant regard to the quality of life. Treatment has to be interpreted as that which is in the best interests of the patient; this may mean settling for comfort. Treatment depends upon judgement not absolutes.

West (1978) comments that in terminal-care situations, the physiotherapist has two goals: the maintenance or restoration of the patient's physical independence and the prevention of deformities that may curtail independence. Keeping a patient mobile and independent helps raise self-respect. It is irrelevant that this independence may not be long-lasting; at the terminal phase of life, achievement lost or gained is viewed on a day-to-day basis. Deformities cause unnecessary stress and discomfort that may make the last weeks of a patient's life a time of increasingly painful dependence. Skilful use of drugs will relieve pain in such a way that the patient may remain mentally alert. A physiotherapist can often continue her work well into the terminal phase of illness.

Some patients find massage a help; it is not an old-fashioned mode of care, but helps to ease pain through the sense of touch. Touch is very important to a person in the last stages of life; it is also a chance for patients to talk. A prerequisite of care is the ability to give time — time to listen and time to offer support. Simple measures such as vibrations may loosen secretions and encouragement to take a few extra deep breaths can relieve distress.

Relatives need support and advice. If a patient is to be nursed at home, relatives have to be shown how to offer understanding and help. For example, they may need to be shown how to move a painful limb correctly. Such help will alleviate feelings of inadequacy and despair.

Kubler-Ross (1970) recognised five stages that patients pass through before accepting the finality of imminent death: denial, anger, bargaining, depression and acceptance. These are normal reactions to an unpleasant truth. The stages are not always clear cut and each patient will react differently. The physiotherapist must recognise the stages and take them as they come, adapting care accordingly, adjusting the approach to suit the needs of particular patients. Therapy given to a dying elderly patient is not a waste of time. Any care that helps the patient to accept his dying and ease his physical discomfort should be given without hesitation.

The physiotherapist will also see relatives after the death of patients. She can be of assistance in helping relatives to cope with the shock of a final diagnosis or with immediate grief reactions. Communication with the recent bereaved is difficult and not a time to impart information, as it is unlikely to be remembered. People need time to grieve and time to be free from invasive 'helpers'. There is a tendency either to weep or to talk and both must be permitted. Bereavement may mean a loss of economic status — giving up a home, moving to a new unfamiliar environment, the problem of loneliness and learning to cope alone. The elderly are also prone to serious illness during bereavement, so it is a time when they are particularly at risk.

Bereavement brings about a crisis of loss, probably the most severe crisis in human existence. For elderly mourners, long, supportive contact and counselling is required. Once a trusting relationship has been established, other helpers may be included. The widening of contact can help to avoid a degree of dependence. The physiotherapist should be aware of such dependence as it is a common feature in the treatment of the older patient. All physiotherapists have to face the dilemma of terminating a course of treatment. There is the risk of throwing the mourner back into the original grief situation at the threat of termination of care, or when the individual trusted helper is not available.

Most people are only intimately concerned with death a few times in their lives. Then it is a major event and time should be left for them to adjust to it. However, the physiotherapist working with the elderly may be faced with several deaths in a year. They may lose patients whom they have come to know over a long time and this may be especially saddening. Any contact with someone who is dying inevitably awakens some personal response. Either acceptance or attempts to suppress feelings can be stressful. This may lead to fatigue, overactivity and irritability. These may jeopardise effectiveness at work and also interfere with personal and family life.

Putting ourselves imaginatively in another's place can increase sensitivity to their needs and can help in deciding what would be best for them. It can also lead to serious mistakes if one does not take into account the fact that one can never fully know what it is like to be the other person. Such a danger is very real for the young physiotherapist attempting to identify with an elderly patient. There is the danger of over-involvement. It is important that the physiotherapist does not permit herself to get into the position of feeling the patient to be her own mother or grandmother. The physiotherapist should cultivate interests quite separate from her professional life. The more a person learns to shed her concern for her patients when she is not at work, the more deeply she can allow herself to be involved when she is at work. Alternative ways of coping by denial, suppression or becoming hardened may be just as costly in the end.

One of the dangers of over-involvement is that the physiotherapist may suddenly become aloof in an effort to create professional detachment and this ultimately denies the patient an essential part of care. Avoidance of the issue can be seen in all members of the caring team. Physiotherapists have a tendency to maintain a brusque cheerfulness, concentrating on solving practical problems and finding different ways of being too busy to spend much time with the dying patient.

Certain mental mechanisms used by patients can cause undue stress to staff if they are not recognised and acknowledged. The two most important are displacement and projection. Displacement is disturbing when the patient's anger about impending death is directed at staff who are accused, for example, of lack of care. It is important that the physiotherapist, at whom such comments may be directed, does not take them personally. Projection may occur when the patient or relative cannot tolerate the knowledge of impending death and projects it onto others. They may say distressing things like, 'Your treatment is killing me'. If projection is not understood, the physiotherapist may begin to doubt if she is doing the right thing by continuing treatment. If the patient should die shortly after treatment, the physiotherapist may become distressed. Inexperienced staff need support in these circumstances.

If there is unsatisfactory communication between a doctor and the patient or relatives, rather than resort to guessing games and subterfuges, many patients or their relatives turn to other members of staff for information regarding their condition. Some patients do so by choice, perhaps intimidated by the consultant and his retinue. They feel more comfortable and at ease asking the physiotherapist during treatment. Providing there is a team policy, this can be satisfactory and the patient will get the information required. If there is no clear policy, then the patient or relative asking the questions may get no answer or an evasive response, or a quick unfounded reassurance or just an embarrassed reaction. These reactions may be taken as meaning that the right answer is too painful, so the patient remains in ignorance but more frightened than before.

Stedford (1984) suggests that poor communication about illness causes more suffering than any other problem, except that of unrelieved pain. When things go wrong, it is often claimed that lack of time and poor working conditions are contributing causes. This may be so, but insensitivity, a reluctance on the part of the staff themselves to face issues and ignorance are causes too.

REFERENCES

Charleton, J.W. and Coles, M.P. (1982) 'Care of the dying.' In D. Coakley and V.J. Hanson (eds), *Nursing and the doctor*, Pitman, London

Kubler-Ross, E. (1970) *On Death and Dying*. Macmillan Co., New York

Stedford, A. (1984) *Facing death. Patients, families and professionals*. William Heinemann Medical Books, London

West, B. (1978) 'In-patient management in a hospice.' In C.M. Saunders (ed), *The management of terminal disease*, Edward Arnold, London and Baltimore

14

Hospital and Community Services

Since World War II, dramatic changes have occurred in the care of elderly people in western societies. The custodial approach inherited from the workhouse period gradually changed and more emphasis was placed on the correct assessment of elderly patients, followed by appropriate treatment and care. The importance of a team approach to treatment was recognised and more and more elderly people were discharged from hospital to their own homes. Emphasis was placed on the alternative of day care and a concerted effort was made to develop resources in the community

During this period of development, geriatric medicine grew as a specialty and it acted as a catalyst for other areas of growth. The geriatric department in most areas played a central role in the services for the elderly. In the British Isles the majority of departments of geriatric medicine have assessment, rehabilitation and long-stay wards. However, this pattern is not universal and in some areas, all patients of different categories are treated in the same ward.

WARD UNITS

The assessment unit in the hospital may be defined as an area in a general hospital that can offer total investigative, consultative and therapeutic services for patients aged 65 and over. The unit is under the control of the consultant physician in geriatric medicine. There are three main identifiable areas in the work of a geriatric assessment unit: diagnosis, treatment and initiation of rehabilitation. A thorough medical investigation is carried out and appropriate treatment is prescribed. Many of the patients are acutely ill on admission.

The multidisciplinary team is involved in the initial assessment of the patient and a clinical management programme is planned. Many of the patients go home directly from the unit or to appropriate community accommodation. Some patients will need a longer period of rehabilitation and these may be transferred to a rehabilitation unit.

The patients requiring physical rehabilitation are predominantly suffering from stroke, parkinsonism and arthritis, together with those recovering from fractures. At the end of the rehabilitation period, most patients return to the community. However, some patients will remain severely handicapped and will need continuing nursing care. These patients are usually transferred to extended-care or long-term-care wards. Extended-care nursing, therefore, is concerned with persons who are no longer capable of meeting their own basic needs. These patients usually need maintenance physiotherapy, as otherwise they will deteriorate further and develop contractures and other complications. Physiotherapists may delegate some of these functions to other staff, but it is important that physiotherapists in a geriatric department should be involved and make a contribution to the quality of care in the extended-care section of the department. A minority of patients from these extended-care units may go home eventually. Quality of life for the patient is important in all parts of the geriatric department. However, it is particularly relevant in the extended-care areas, where these wards literally become the home of the patient. All members of the geriatric team should be interested in seeing that the quality of care is as good as possible. Go-ahead units have achieved encouraging results by using music and art in long-term care units (Denham 1983).

DAY HOSPITAL

The day hospital may be defined as a place having the facilities to provide services for patients without admitting them as in-patients. It does not, therefore, have an independent existence, but is simply an extension of the service provided in hospital, so that patients who are not resident in the hospital can benefit from its services. If it is situated on the site of a general hospital, the day hospital may provide a full assessment service. This may also obviate the need for hospital admission in the first instance. However, rehabilitation is the dominant function of most day hospitals.

Some day hospitals maintain patients who are heavily disabled after discharge. By bringing such patients to the day hospital, maybe once a week, it not only enables the patient to benefit from physiotherapy, but also gives a caring family a much needed break. An important benefit of the day hospital is that it preserves the patient's links with the community. Frequency of attendance at the day hospital will vary, depending upon individual circumstances. The period of treatment will also vary with each patient. However, if the day hospital is to work successfully, each patient must have an individual treatment plan designed by the clinical team. There must also be regular reviews of patients and regular discharges. Apart from giving individual therapy, physiotherapists usually organise group therapy at the day hospital. In some areas, links with the community are strengthened further by the development of community physiotherapy services.

LINKS WITH THE COMMUNITY

Most departments of geriatric medicine have strong links with the community. Pre-admission assessment is often carried out in the patient's home. This helps the clinical team in forming their treatment plan. If there is a waiting list for admission, it also helps to set an order of priority. In many units, these assessment visits are carried out by a doctor, but it has been shown by Pathy, Hughes and White (1972) that an equally objective assessment may be carried out by a properly trained health visitor attached to the geriatric unit. In most departments of geriatric medicine, liaison health visitors and community nurses attend the discharge conferences. This allows the smooth transition of the patient from hospital to the home setting. Members of the rehabilitation team may visit the patient's home before discharge, often taking the patient with them so they can assess his performance in the home setting. Trial discharge for high-risk patients is a useful way of ascertaining whether the patient will be able to cope at home. The patient's bed is kept reserved for him for a few days after discharge, in case the situation proves non-viable. Trial discharges must involve close co-operation between the hospital and the community teams.

INTERMITTENT RELIEF ADMISSIONS

Some patients remain severely incapacitated even after physiotherapy.

These patients may be suitable for a long-term, nursing-care unit, but caring relatives may be anxious to try and cope at home. Many departments of geriatric medicine have a facility that enables such patients to be admitted intermittently to hospital from home. The period between admissions and the length of the admission will depend on the individual case. Using a hospital bed in this manner is a sensible use of a scarce resource, as it benefits more than one patient and family. Families who are prepared to care for heavily dependent relatives should be helped in every way possible. The policy, which provides annual holiday relief by admitting a heavily dependent old person for a short period so that the relatives can go away, is usually greatly appreciated.

SPECIAL UNITS

The scope of geriatric medicine is so great that it was inevitable that special units should develop to cope with particular problems. Such special services include incontinence clinics, limb-amputee clinics, stroke units, psychogeriatric assessment units and joint orthopaedic/geriatric medicine units. Effective incontinence clinics involve co-operation between the geriatrician, urologist and gynaecologist. Many of the patients undergoing orthopaedic surgery are frail and elderly. Best results are achieved when elderly patients are properly assessed and medically treated, when necessary, before operation. Early pre- and post-operative collaborative involvement between the departments of geriatric medicine and orthopaedics considerably improves the overall management of the older patient with a fracture.

Stroke units have been developed to deal specifically with the rehabilitation of the stroke patient. Isaacs, Neville and Rushford (1976) found that one-third of the patients referred to a stroke unit in Glasgow were under the age of 65, one-third were aged between 65 and 74 and one-third were aged 75 and over. Kennedy (1976) considered that stroke units were most appropriately located within a department of geriatric medicine.

COMMUNITY SERVICES

The purpose of community services for the elderly is to make it possible for people to continue to live in their own homes and to participate as fully as possible in community activities throughout old age. This benefits not only the individual but also the community, because of the soaring costs of institutional care. Since its inception, the National Health Service in the United Kingdom has placed emphasis on the development of community services. There is therefore a comprehensive network of facilities available in many districts and these are funded by the State.

Considerable good work is also being carried out by voluntary bodies such as Age Concern, an organisation that has prompted the welfare of the elderly in Britain over the past 40 years. This body is involved in various practical programmes, information services, training programmes and research projects. It has an invaluable publication section for anyone involved in services for older people (Age Concern 1980). There are many other voluntary bodies involved with the elderly and the physiotherapist should know of the voluntary bodies in her own area as they may have very important contributions to make to the overall welfare of patients.

Good neighbours, family and friends can provide many of the services that an older person needs to stay independent in the community. However, when a patient is severely disabled, even the most caring families will need support. The less severely handicapped may require support if there is not a caring family network around them. Careful assessment of each individual should determine which services are appropriate. The physiotherapist and occupational therapist play key roles in assessing the needs of the patient. It is a mistake to consider it solely the function of a social worker. The nature of services available vary from locality to locality, but certain basic services are available in most areas.

THE GENERAL PRACTITIONER AND DOMICILLARY NURSE

The general practitioner (family doctor) is responsible for the primary care of the older person in the community. He is the leader of the health-care team covering his patients (primary health-care team). The community team includes the nurse, the physiotherapist, the occupational therapist and the social worker. In Ireland, the community nurse is known as the public health nurse. In the British system, community nursing is divided into two main subgroups — the health visitor and the district nurse. The district nurse carries out nursing routines in the home and the health visitor concentrates on health education. The ability to shift emphasis from the institution to community care in the area depends to a very large extent on the nursing facilities available. For instance, it is not possible to maintain a person who needs regular nursing care in the home unless a night-nursing service is available.

A health visitor is a nurse with a post-registration qualification, a health visitor's certificate. She can play an important role in changing negative attitudes towards the problems of ageing and she can also bring elderly people in the community with a treatable condition to the attention of the doctor and other members of the primary health-care team. In certain areas, a number of health visitors specialise particularly in problems of elderly patients.

THE OCCUPATIONAL THERAPIST

The occupational therapist plays an important role in assessing the patient in his home. She can advise the family or patient on how best they might cope and she can provide any aids and equipment that might be necessary. Apart from aids, the home of an elderly patient may need adaptation. For instance, grab rails may be needed in the toilet or bathroom; additional rails may be needed on the stairs. Doors may need to be widened or ramps installed for a wheelchair. In carrying out assessments of this nature, it is most useful if the occupational therapist and the physiotherapist visit the house together.

COMMUNITY PHYSIOTHERAPIST

In the community the physiotherapist has educational as well as rehabilitative functions. At the present time, rehabilitation services primarily take place within the hospital, or in a hospital-based environment. Though provision of service in the community is advancing, it is doing so at an alarmingly slow pace. A number of physiotherapy schemes run from local health centres are very successful. Often treatment may be offered to a patient more quickly than if he had to wait for out-patient care or admission.

One of the objections to a comprehensive community physiotherapy scheme is that it is not cost-effective: little heed is paid to a patient's needs or requirements. In the UK the publication of the Tunbridge (1972) sub-committee report supported such a viewpoint. However, Frazer (1981) has shown that a domicillary physiotherapist working in the community can maintain a list of about 24 patients each week. Some patients will require daily care, whereas others will be maintained at home by a visit once a week or less often.

Frazer (1982) divided the treatment used in the community into six separate categories:

1. Advice and management instruction, common to most treatments;
2. Exercise, massage, mobilisation, postural drainage [no equipment required];
3. Heat and cold applications;
4. Ultrasound, low- and medium-frequency currents [special equipment required];
5. Intermittent positive-pressure ventilation, suction;
6. Traction [not likely for the older patient].

The equipment required is, on the whole, portable. Results obtained are the same, whether carried out in a hospital or at home. The physiotherapist working in the community can have access to small equipment (balls, quoits, bands, etc.) and aids for the activities of daily living.

Naturally, transport of some kind is required for a physiotherapist working in people's homes. If their own transport is used, then appropriate mileage allowances must be met by the authorities responsible for the overall organisation of the service. It is claimed by some that the physiotherapists in the community spend their day travelling in a car and little time is spent with the patient. The amount of time spent 'on the road' will vary from area to area and from urban to rural districts. Minimum time spent travelling is achieved through sensible overall planning of the service and individual planning and organisation of the day's programme.

Different attitudes are required for work within the community. An obvious difference is that the physiotherapist is on her own and is a visitor to the patient's home. The normal back-up facilities available in a hospital are not readily and immediately available in the home setting. The physiotherapist must be aware of the resources and personnel available within her area of cover. There may be resentment at the physiotherapist's presence in the home and the creation of a feeling of inadequacy on the part of relatives. It is very important to make relatives, or friends and neighbours if appropriate, a part of the treatment programme so that they will gradually take over the treatment. It is more difficult to terminate a treatment programme in someone's home surroundings; such termination requires understanding, sympathy and above all, the preparation of both the patient and his relatives and friends.

Frazer (1982) summarised physiotherapy in the community as follows:

1. Many of the disabilities of patients referred to the service can be alleviated by appropriate physiotherapy;
2. Domicillary physiotherapy service is an effective way to provide treatment for the patient who is unable to travel independently to hospital;
3. There is a minimum of equipment required to provide a domicillary service;
4. The patient's relatives are able to provide considerable help at no cost to the State;
5. The involvement of relatives in the day-to-day treatment of the patient can reduce the number of visits that need to be made by the physiotherapist;
6. The involvement of relatives with physiotherapists has increased public awareness of the significance of physiotherapy;
7. Patients who previously would have been denied physiotherapy treatment will have access to such care;
8. Rehabilitation can be provided within the patient's home without the need for expensive ambulance services;
9. In certain cases, hospital admission may be avoided;
10. Treatment given in the home is relevant both to the patient and his relatives; it involves him in little inconvenience, no discomfort and minimal strain.

SOCIAL WORKERS

Despite efforts to educate elderly people about entitlements to various services and benefits there is still a lack of understanding amongst many about these matters. Social workers play an important role in the community in mobilising the services that are available for the elderly. They also assist elderly people with problems of isolation and loneliness. By arranging support services, they can prevent the unnecessary admission of a patient. When care of an institutional nature is absolutely necessary, they can acquaint the patient with the options available and help to make appropriate arrangements.

CHIROPODY

Foot ailments are among the main reasons why an old person becomes housebound and immobile. A domicillary service is therefore very important.

SPEECH THERAPY

The speech-therapy services are particularly important for people who have suffered a stroke. Most areas do not have an adequate number of speech therapists working in the community. The volunteer stroke scheme is active in some areas (see Chapter 5).

HOME-HELP SERVICES

The home-help service is designed to assist people with household duties and personal care that they cannot cope with themselves and which relatives and friends are either unwilling or unable to perform for them. The service generally involves one to three hours per day for a number of days per week, depending upon individual needs.

MEALS-ON-WHEELS

This service provides meals for persons who are unable to cook regular meals for themselves and who cannot get meals from any other source. Most recipients of meals-on-wheels are elderly. It is particularly important for older patients who are nutritionally at risk.

DAY CENTRES

Luncheon clubs have been developed in some areas as a facility for the elderly. This provides both nutrition and social contact. A day centre is a more 'supportive' facility as it provides partial or complete day care. A day centre provides lunch and also offers a selection of activities. It may offer chiropody, hair-dressing and baths. Adequate day-care facilities make the management of the dependent elderly-at-home much easier for both the family and the community care team. Day-care centres are also essential if the day hospital is to function properly as otherwise the day hospital will gradually accumulate a large number of people who are attending solely for social reasons. Unlike day hospitals, day centres do not provide medical investigation or treatment facilities. However, some day centres have physiotherapy facilities and this is an opportunity to maintain those who attend at their maximum function.

SHELTERED HOUSING AND RESIDENTIAL CARE

Sheltered housing offers an alternative to full residential or hospital care when disability is not very severe. Sheltered housing exists in many forms and has proven to be a very effective method of keeping elderly people in the community. It consists of self-contained living units grouped together and there is usually a resident warden or supervisor. There is not enough sheltered housing available and because of this, many elderly people have to apply for full residential care.

Residential care (welfare homes) provides institutional accommodation for elderly people who are frail but ambulant, continent and mentally clear and not in need of continuing nursing care. In recent years, special residential care facilities have been developed for the mentally confused elderly. These are known as elderly-mentally-infirm (EMI) homes. Welfare homes become more difficult to manage if the residents become immobile. For this reason, in some areas, physiotherapists visit welfare homes regularly to ensure that any mobility problems are identified early and dealt with appropriately. Physiotherapists should also have a role in educating the elderly residents about ways of keeping active (see Chapter 11) and likewise, educating the officers running these homes. Unfortunately, it has been found that the regime in many residential homes makes residents increasingly dependent and eventually unwilling to do things for themselves (Gibberd 1977).

PRIVATE NURSING HOMES

In recent years, there has been a growth in the number of private nursing homes for elderly people in the United Kingdom and Ireland. Many similar homes exist in the United States and other countries. Patients in many of these homes are supported by supplements from the State. The majority of residents in most of the homes are ambulant. However, some homes do provide nursing care for heavily dependent patients and these homes tend to be more expensive. All of these institutions have to meet certain basic standards before they are officially approved.

REFERENCES

Age Concern (1980) *Age concern at work*, Age Concern, London

Denham, M.J. (1983) *Care of the long-stay elderly patient*. Croom Helm, London

Frazer, F.W. (1981) 'Domicillary physiotherapy: cost and benefit,' PhD Thesis, University of Aston

—— (1982) 'Physiotherapy in the community.' In F.W. Frazer (ed), *Rehabilitation within the community*, Faber and Faber, London

Gibberd, K. (1977) *Home for life. What alternatives*? Age Concern, London

Isaacs, B., Neville, T. and Rushford, I. (1976) 'The stricken — the social consequence of a stroke.' *Age and Ageing, 5*, 188

Kennedy, B.F. (1976) 'The stroke unit — a physiotherapist's views.' *Physiotherapy, 62*, 5, 154–53

Pathy, M.S., Hughes, J.N.P. and White, W.M. (1972) 'The role of the specialist health visitor in the geriatric team.' *Community Med., 15*, 206

Tunbridge Report (1972) 'Rehabilitation.' A report of a sub-committee of the standing medical advisory committee. HMSO, London

15

Aids, Equipment and Appliances

Nichols and Williams (1977) define an 'aid' as a small, easily handled device that will improve a patient's functional capability. If this goal necessitates a large, bulky or non-portable device, the word 'equipment' is used. If the device is purposefully made to fit an individual it becomes an 'appliance'.

Whether it is deemed suitable for a patient to have an aid, some equipment or an appliance, the essential requirements are that:

1. The patient must need the aid in order to assist independence;
2. The aid must serve that need;
3. The aid must be made of standard components and be pleasant to look at;
4. The aid must be mechanically dependable, cheap and durable;
5. The aid must be simple to manage.

Many devices may be mass-produced, but some will have to be tailor-made for the patient; this is especially true of splints. If a splint is to serve its purpose, then it must be individually made.

There are several booklets that may be of great help to both the older person and to relatives and friends. In most countries, health authorities and government agencies produce booklets that describe the entitlements of the elderly — cheap fuel schemes; dental services; disability benefits; health services; laundry services; library services; legal aid; maintenance allowances; meals-on-wheels; pensions; travel schemes, etc. There are several books on the theme of 'Guide for the Disabled', which give much information of value to the older person. There are many inexpensive booklets on cooking and gardening for the older patient.

WALKING AIDS

Bruell and Peszczynski (1958) consider that the ability to move about on one's own is a prerequisite to independence. Aids that may assist elderly people range from the simple to the complex, depending on the problem to be solved or overcome. The appropriate aid should be individually selected and the patient should be instructed adequately in its use. An unsuitable aid can hinder progress and be dangerous. The elderly patient must be advised not to borrow another person's aid and not to use a husband's or wife's temporarily. The patient must have confidence in any helper, so an assistant must be shown how to give effective and safe assistance. The usual fault is for someone to offer more physical support than is necessary. This disturbs the normal rhythm of movement and so makes walking more difficult.

Walking aids must have a ferrule of at least a 3.0 cm in diameter: these must not be worn or dirty and the patient should be advised to rotate the ferrule regularly to achieve even wear. The patient must have the dangers of worn and dirty ferrules clearly explained. Ice-gripping ferrules are also available. There is a tendency to think of a stick as always having a C-shaped handle, because that is the handle that most manufacturers produce. However, for many patients it is not suitable. Plastazote or similar material may be used to hand-mould the handle. One of the most frequent problems for anyone using a stick, but especially for the elderly, is where to put it when not in use; a leather thong attached to the handle of the stick or an elastic loop around the handle plus a larger loop around the wrist, leaves the hand free to grasp a doorknob or railing. This can be a difficult manoeuvre for the arthritic, who often hang the C-shaped handle over the arm. The patient must be warned not to let a 'dangling' stick get caught in stair rods or stair rails, or between their own legs. A useful tip is to keep a spare stick at the top of a set of stairs.

Elbow crutches, gutter crutches, axillary crutches, walking frames, rollators, quadrupods and so on may be provided as and when necessary and when suitable for specific conditions. Accurate measurement of all aids is essential. Walking frames take up a lot of room and often encourage instability of gait. The patient frequently walks too far into the frame, thus throwing balance backwards. This can occur even after careful instructions. However, the walking frame is a useful aid for some elderly people and is their sole means of mobility. Patients who tend to fall backwards or those

Figure 15.1: Toe raising caliper

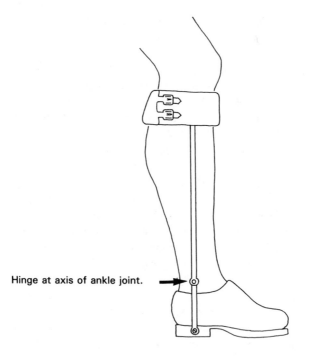

Hinge at axis of ankle joint.

with an ataxic gait may be helped if the frame is weighted. Marks halfway along the sides of the frame can help indicate how far into the frame the patient should walk, though it encourages the patient to look at the floor rather than straight ahead.

It should be remembered that in the home, a tea trolley functions both as an aid to walking and as a method of carrying objects around. When advising purchase, it must be strong enough and balanced so that it can be leant on without tipping; ideally it should be fitted with 'Shepherd' castors for easy moving and steering.

When prescribing an aid, knowledge of the environment in which it is to be used is essential, for example, the size of doorways, the number of steps and stairs, the turns on stairs, the type of furniture and the floor surface. The physiotherapist must ensure that the patient will be able to cope with all likely demands.

The provision of a shoe raise, surgical shoes or splints may help some patients to walk. These must be individually made. The reason that so many toe-raising devices are a failure and why so many patients are reluctant to wear them, is that they do not help walking. They are mechanically unsound and often work against the patient. The aid must mechanically assist and mimic the events at the ankle that are involved in walking. The joint of the caliper must be on a level with and in line with the ankle joint, where dorsiflexion and plantarflexion occur. The caliper must enter the shoe perpendicularly below the joint (see Fig. 15.1). A cheap, effective and unobtrusive way of helping a patient who has an unstable ankle and a foot that supinates is to ask him to wear shoes with flared heels.

Parallel bars

Parallel bars of adequate length and complete stability are essential in any physiotherapy department that treats elderly patients. A minimum length of 8–10 m (25–30 ft) is desirable to allow for a reasonable walk; the height should be around 88 cm (34.5 in) and the width 58.4–61 cm (23–4 in) (Finlay 1981). The bars should be positioned away from the wall so that the physiotherapist can walk with the patient on either side if necessary. At each end of the parallel bars there must be sufficient space to permit easy manipulation of wheelchairs.

COMMUNICATION

The life of the older person can often be lonely; aids which assist effective communication are an advantage to both the patient and to those around them. There are adaptations for telephones and sophisticated intercom devices on the market, which also give the patient confidence and ease the fears associated with living alone.

Reading aids

There is an abundance of aids on the market that enable frail people to hold reading matter and turn pages if required. Those with unsteady or weak hands may turn a page using a rubber thimble. As eye sight fails, a magnifying glass is of help, but equally, a patient should be advised on adequate illumination. Talking books are available as are large-print editions of many books and some magazines.

Writing aids

Patients may be advised about writing at a table of the correct height; this should permit complete forearm support at all times. The use of larger sheets of paper, in a block or fixed to a clipboard, make life somewhat easier. Felt tip pens are easier to write with than other materials and there are pen holders and paintbrush holders on the market which increase the diameter of the pen. Ultralite 'finger yokes' help to stabilise the forefinger when gripping a pen, pencil or brush.

Telephone aids

The telephone has become a vital form of communication and should be available to all who live alone. Advances in technology have produced an exciting range of adaptations that help the caller to dial and call numbers, to use the telephone and to hear incoming calls. The patient can speak into microphones and receive answers via a loudspeaker; punch cards will dial numbers and push-button telephones are easier to manage than dial phones. Advice can be given to the elderly about the positioning of the telephone, extensions or cordless phones, especially if mobility is impaired.

THE HOME

Often minor modifications to the home can minimise hazards yet improve independence. A few steps, or even one steep step at the entrance to a house or flat can imprison the elderly. The height of a step may be reduced by the addition of a half-step. A ramp may replace a step, but the rate of the raise should be no more than 30 cm (11.8 in) in 360 cm (141.7 in); this is often not practical. Rails may be fitted if absent. Surfaces of steps and ramps should be non-slip.

Doors

If gripping a door handle or holding a key is a difficulty, there are many useful devices on the market, such as door-knob levers and levering handles. Key holders are made in many styles. Simple ideas that will increase the leverage may be introduced by having a metal plate riveted to a key, or by putting a piece of dowelling through the hole in a key, or by fitting the key into a slit in a wooden block and securing it with a screw.

Floors

Floor surfaces and covering should be kept in good repair; frayed carpets, loose tiles, scatter rugs and glazed tiles are common causes of accidents. During rehabilitation, patients should attempt activities on a variety of floor surfaces and particularly on surfaces to be coped with in and around the home. It must not be forgotten that few homes have the absolutely level linoleum and polished wood surfaces that are so often found in the hospital setting.

Lighting and electricity

Many elderly people have either a fear of, or a blind faith in, electricity. Sockets should be positioned so that stooping is minimised (40 cm (15.6 in) from the floor). Rocker-action light switches require little pressure to activate. Trailing wires in a house are a danger, yet are all too common in do-it-yourself jobs.

Hand reachers

There are many hand-reachers available to enable the older person to get something that is just out of reach. Many of these devices have magnets attached to them for picking up pins, clips, etc. They come in different weights and lengths and some are designed so that they fold away.

Furniture

Muston *et al.* (1981) have shown that elderly people are likely to find getting out of a chair difficult. In a survey, 42 per cent of patients experienced difficulty in rising from a chair and 34 per cent experienced discomfort. He concluded that chairs that are easy to get out of are essential. Older people take longer to get out of a chair.

They tend to rely on hand grips for balance and they recruit thrust from arm as well as leg muscles. Choosing appropriate furniture is important and there are three criteria: comfort, mobility and safety. Many old people like a footstool, yet it is a hazard as it is easy to trip over one. It is recommended that a gap of 20 cm (7.9 in) should separate a chair seat and the underside of a table. Finlay *et al.* (1983) found that ambulant residents with moderate or serious difficulty in rising could get up most easily from a seat height of 40.6–43.2 cm (16–17 in) and also that arms positioned at least 25.4 cm (10 in) above the seat height gave the greatest advantage. The physiotherapist should ensure that the department has a wide range of chairs of different heights. Chairs are now available in which the height is adjustable and the angle of the seat can be altered.

The bedroom

Modern beds are usually between 38–55 cm (15–21.6 in) high. In order to transfer from a chair to a bed, the heights must be approximately the same (about 47 cm [18.5 in]), so the bed may need to be lowered or raised on blocks. In hospital all beds should be adjustable in order to facilitate transfer from the bed to a chair, commode, etc. A safe braking-system is essential. Andrews and Atkinson (1982) give practical advice on important aspects of equipping wards and units for elderly patients.

For the older person, special attention should be paid to the protection of the skin. The ideal mattress is a Polyfloat mattress (the upper layer being cut in order to form a number of almost independent blocks) with a soft, loose-fitting mattress cover. Many items other than beds have been designed to prevent pressure sores: cushions, ripple beds, sheepskin rugs, and so on (see Chapter 9). The freedom that a duvet offers is an asset in reducing the likelihood of flexion contractures at the ankle and it also makes it easier for the patient to turn frequently. Some patients require a bed cradle. However, these tend to be bulky and patients often complain of feeling cold.

Hoists are generally recommended not so much as an aid for the independence, comfort and safety of the elderly patient, but for the assistance of a helper (Haworth and Nichols 1980). There are many types of hoist available and selection will depend upon individual circumstances (portable hydraulic; fixed electric; electric on a ceiling-mounted track).

The bathroom

Many more elderly people could use a lavatory if it were the correct height and if grab rails were suitably placed around it. A seat-rise of between 8–15 cm (3–6 in) is normally required. Such seat-rises are available in one-piece mouldings of high-density plastic, which are totally watertight. The height and spacing of grab rails is of considerable importance and can only be determined by trial. A bottom wiper that enables the user to clean from the front is now available. This restores dignity and privacy to an important aspect of normal hygiene.

Bathing can be made easier by having shallow baths, sit-in baths, bath cabinets, etc., but all these devices are expensive and require extensive alterations. Baths with an adjustable height are now available on the market to allow easier management and transfer of patients. In the home, simple devices are usually employed to make bathing easier and safer and include bath boards, grab rails, and non-slip mats. Bath seats need to be designed on an individual basis. The usual method of standing on one leg to get into and out of the bath is potentially dangerous for the elderly. By sitting on a stool or board, the legs can be swung over the bath edge and access is very much easier. Chamberlain *et al.* (1981) have shown that accidents may occur if the boards are fixed too high or move during use. Sideways-wedging bath seats are unsuitable for acrylic baths as they might split the bath. On the whole, the design of bath boards is unsuitable as they are too narrow and usually covered with an inappropriate surface. Chamberlain *et al.* have also shown that such aids should be obtained from the hospital and that early instruction in their use at home should be given by the therapist. Follow-up instruction should be given at home on one or two occasions, as this results in a great increase in confidence.

Other accessories include bath mats with rubber grips, magnetic soap-holders, suction-type soap-holders, non-slip strips for the bath and shower and folding shower-seats. Showers are not yet favoured by many elderly people, but used with a shower chair, they may in fact be very suitable for some. Showers should have controls that are accessible to a helper; the shower head should be fixed, but should have several different positions.

The kitchen

The elderly require a kitchen where appliances, provisions and cooking utensils are stored near their place of use and within easy reach. Work surfaces, where possible, may be adapted so that the individual can work from a chair. Cutlery comes in many ranges: there are right- and left-handed knives, forks and spoons; padded handles; ultra-light knives, forks and spoons; scissors that operate by a squeezing action. Knives are designed with the handle at right angles to the blade so that the cutting power from the arm is transferred to the centre of the blade. The classic design 'Nelson' knife is available for one-handed eating.

Non-slip materials that do not stick to a surface can keep plates steady and act as a grip for opening jars and so on. Other kitchen devices for the elderly are kettle tippers, teapot stands, breadboards with spikes, potato peelers, bottle stands, left- and right-handed can openers; tap-turners and bendistraws. Household chores can be aided by lightweight, easy-to-move pails, long-handled dust mops, cellulose sponge mops and non-stoop dustpans.

The stairs

Between 13 and 25 per cent of accidental falls at home occur on the stairs. However, following a fall anywhere in the home, many elderly people are afraid of using the stairs. Double handrails greatly improve the confidence of some patients. Hospital stairs are often unsuitable for stair practice because of incorrect width, too steep a gradient or unsuitable hand rails. Finlay (1983) has recommended that each physiotherapy department dealing with the elderly should construct a set of practice stairs and institute a stair-training programme.

DRESSING AND PERSONAL CARE

Washing parts of the body is made easier by long-handled brushes and sponges; soap on a rope is useful in a bath or shower. Some people find it easier to use a mitt rather than a face flannel. Mitts are made in a variety of materials including sponge. Handles of toothbrushes can be built up in the same way as eating utensils; some patients find an electric toothbrush easier to use, since the handle is larger and less wrist and arm movement is necessary.

The elderly should be encouraged to use an electric razor, but shaving is a very personal event, so handles of safety razors may be adapted if necessary. Older people find toenails difficult to cut and chiropody services are often needed. Finger nails should be kept clean and short especially in those patients with poor peripheral circulation.

Clothing for the upper part of the body should, whenever possible, fasten at the front; zips may be modified by inserting a curtain ring through the eyelet of the pull tag for a better grip. Buttons may be replaced by Velcro. Trousers are in many ways more sensible than skirts, tights and stockings; they are easier to put on, warmer and may hide callipers, splints or artificial limbs. Devices such as long-handled shoehorns, stocking aids, tights aids and support stockings are available, together with dressing sticks and elastic laces.

It is important to encourage the patient to do as much as possible without reliance on aids. Cluttering a patient's life with aids can, ironically, produce the reverse effect to that required and induce a sense of dependence and apathy. Attitudes are more important than appliances. However, when used judiciously, they have a place. They should only be given after a very careful assessment and the use made of the aid by the patient should be monitored regularly.

REFERENCES

Andrews, J. and Atkinson, L. (1982) 'Ward furniture, equipment and patient clothing.' In D. Coakley (ed), *Establishing a geriatric service*, Croom Helm, London

Bruell, J.H. and Peszczynski, M. (1958) 'Perception of verticality in hemiplegic patients in relation to rehabilitation.' *Clin. Orthop., 12*, 124

Chamberlain, M.A., Thornley, G., Stow, J. and Wright, V. (1981) 'Evaluation of aids and equipment for the bath.' *Rheumatol. and Rehab., 20*, 38

Finlay, O. (1981) 'Functional research project — parallel bars specifically for the elderly.' *Abstracts, 2*, 3, 5–9

——— Bayles, T.B., Rosen, C and Milling, J. (1983) 'Effects of chair design, age and cognitive status on mobility.' *Age and the ageing, 12*, 329–35

Haworth, R.J. and Nichols, P.J.R. (1980) 'Hoists in the home; their recommendations and use.' *Rheumatol. and Rehab. 19*, 42

Muston, J.S., Ellis, M., Chamberlain, M. and Wright, V. (1981) 'An investigation into the problems of easy chairs used by the arthritic and elderly.' *Rheumatol. and Rehab., 20*, 164

Nichols, P.J.R. and Williams, E. (1977) 'Aids and appliances.' In S. Mattingly (ed), *Rehabilitation*, Update Books, London

Appendix I

Activities of Daily Living Charts

Dressing

Put on shoes
Fasten shoes
Take off socks/stockings
Put on socks/stockings
Put on corset
Put on bra
Put on pants
Put on garment over feet
Take off garment over feet
Put on garment over head
Take off garment over head

Tie tie
Fasten buttons
Fasten zipper
Fasten hooks
Put on coat
Take off coat
Put on/off gloves
Put on appliance
Take off appliance
Put on splint
Take off splint

Grooming

Comb hair
Wash hair
Clean teeth
Wash face/hands
Dry face/hands

Bath body
Dry body
Turn taps on/off
Shave
Make up face

Feeding

Eat with spoon
Eat with fork

Eat with knife
Drink from cup

Mobility

On/off toilet
On/off commode
In/out bath
On/off chair
In/out bed
Turn in bed
Sit in bed
Balance safely
Stand safely

Walk
Stairs
Propel chair
Transfer to/from chair
Pick up objects from floor/
  table
Carry food on tray
Push trolley
Shopping
In/out car/bus

Communication

Write
Read
Hold/control book
Hold/control paper

Turn television/radio on/off
Hobbies
Light cigarette

Cooking

Lift pans
Fill kettle
Kettle on/off cooker
Turn cooker on/off
Fill teapot
Mix
Pour
Whisk
Cut

Peel
Spread
Put things in/out oven
Light oven
Open jar
Open tins
Slice
Wash/dry dishes
Make pastry

Cleaning

Make bed
Sweep
Dust
Vacuum
Mop
Polish

Clean windows
Wash
Dry
Iron
Shop

General

Open/close doors
Turn key
Draw curtains

Switch on/off light
Put in/pull out plug
Use telephone

(Coates and King 1983)

REFERENCES

Coates, H. and King, A. (1983) *The patient assessment — a handbook for therapists*. Churchill Livingstone, Edinburgh

Appendix II

Suggested Programme of Exercise and Dance

A. In a variety of supported and free positions:

1. Seated on chairs;
2. Standing with chair for support;
3. Free-standing;
4. Moving;
5. Lying on the floor.

B. To music:

1. Varying the beat;
2. Varying the tempo;
3. Adding syncopation;
4. Varying musical selection;
5. Live music.

C. In different combination:

1. Alone;
2. With a partner;
3. In a small group (n = 3–8)
4. As a class (n = up to 20)

D. In different formations:

1. Random arrangements;
2. Circle formation;
3. Line formation.

E. Using different degrees of force:

1. Slow, flowing movements;
2. Quick, staccato movements;
3. Combination of slow and quick movements.

F. Changing body shapes, levels and dimensions:

1. Moving with the body in high space;
2. Moving from one level to another;
3. Making the body small and compact;
4. Stretching the body out to cover maximum space;
5. Moving from one size and shape to another.

G. In different directions

1. Forwards;
2. Backwards;
3. Sideways;
4. Turning;
5. Diagonally.

Appendix III

Suggested Activities Class

1. WARM-UP

A. Spine (seated position)

1. Head circling — clockwise and anticlockwise;
2. Cervical flexion and extension;
3. Cervical rotation — to right and left;
4. Trunk side flexion — to right and left, arms hanging loosely at sides;
5. Extending arms to ceiling and slowly flexing trunk to touch the floor.

B. Shoulder girdle/shoulder/elbow (seated position)

1. Elevation and depression;
2. Retraction and relaxation;
3. Pendular arm swing — flexion and extension;
4. Shoulder abduction and adduction;
5. Alternate hands touching shoulders, circling the elbow;
6. Using a meter stick with fingers flexed and forearm pronated:
    - elbows extended shoulder height — slowly elevating arms above head;
    - elbows extended shoulder height — arms elevated above head — elbows flexed to touch head with stick and elevated again;
    - repeat with elbows flexed and shoulders extended so that the stick is positioned behind head;

— elbows held in extension, stick brought to the vertical position from the horizontal position and vice versa.

C. Wrists/hands (seated position)

1. Starting position, elbows held to waist;
2. Forearm pronation and supination — 'palms up to ceiling and down to floor';
3. Wrist extension and flexion;
4. Wrist circling clockwise and anticlockwise;
5. Making a tight fist and then extending the fingers;
6. Forearms pronated — 'play the piano with your fingers';
7. Wrists relaxed — 'shake your wrists';
8. Fingers extended, abduction and adduction of fingers.

D. Hip/knee/ankle (seated position)

1. Heels on the ground, tapping the toes in time to music;
2. Dorsiflexion and plantarflexion at ankle — lifting the knee off the chair, each time the heel or the toes touch the floor;
3. Extending the knees and pointing the toes;
4. Extending the knees and flexing the hip with knees extended;
5. Hands clasped around alternate knees, flexing the hip and stretching the knee to the chest with hands.

Change to a standing position and

6. Flex alternate knees, standing on the spot (those with aids use them; those with poor balance hold on to the back of a chair);
7. Balancing whilst standing on one foot.

E. End warm-up

Breathing exercises
1. Basal expansion exercise;
2. Diaphragmatic breathing.

2. INDIVIDUAL WORK WITH SMALL BALLS

In a seated position:

1. Bring the ball under alternate legs, lifting the knee off the chair each time;
2. Bring the ball behind the back with the right hand and take it with the left hand and vice versa;
3. Bring the ball behind the head with the right hand and take it in the left hand and vice versa;
4. Using the fingers, move the ball up the arm to the shoulder and down again;
5. With the ball held securely between the ankles, extend the knee to lift the feet off the ground and hold down.

3. GROUP GAMES

1. Patients throwing ball to each other;
2. Patients bouncing ball to each other;
3. Patients kicking ball to each other.

Index